The
Little
Diabetes Book

YOU

Need to Read

Compliments of

ONE TOUCH®
changes everything®

The
Little
Diabetes Book

Need to Read

by
Michael A. Weiss
and Martha M. Funnell

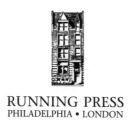

RUNNING PRESS
PHILADELPHIA • LONDON

9 8 7 6 5 4 3 2 1

Library of Congress Cataloging-in-Publication Number:
2007926071

ISBN-13: 978-07624-3022-2
Lifescan California Edition

Cover designed by Bill Jones
Interior designed by Jan Greenberg
Typography: Stone Serif

This book may be ordered by mail from the publisher.
Please include $2.50 for postage and handling.
But try your bookstore first!

Running Press Book Publishers
2300 Chestnut Street
Philadelphia, PA 19103-4371

Visit us on the web!
www.runningpress.com

Dedication

We dedicate this book to our fathers who we lost while writing this book. They taught us to care about others and showed us the strength and courage to try to make a difference.

Table of Contents

Acknowledgments 8
Introduction 11

  1.Who's In Charge? You!......................19
  2. Four LIFE Steps for Living
     with Diabetes.................................29

Part I: Learning
  3. Know Your Opponent 49
  4. Know Your Team 95
  5. Know Yourself.................................119

Part II: Doing
  6. Making Decisions 143
  7. Making Choices...............................165
  8. Making Changes..............................203

Part III: Now What?
  Staying The Course............................225
  Glossary of Terms 245
  Resources...250

Acknowledgments

Our vision for this book is to ease the burden of daily life with diabetes for the millions of people who are affected by it. Our desire to make a difference in the world of diabetes has been a driving force in our volunteer and professional lives for many years.

This book could not have been possible without the continuing collaboration of our friend and colleague, Bob Anderson, at the University of Michigan. Bob's wisdom and spirit, and his incomparable humor, have inspired us throughout this project.

Our friend Larry Kane was an early reader of our manuscript and a major source of encouragement. He has supported our efforts in so many different ways, for which we will always be grateful.

As health professionals, Ann Albright, Davida Kruger, Malinda Peeples, Bob Rakel, Richard Rubin, and Linda Siminerio are respected throughout the world. Each of them is a leader in her or his field, and each read the manuscript, providing us with invaluable insights based on their own experiences. Their patients are truly blessed.

Nicole Johnson, Miss America 1999 and host of MSNBC's d-Life, has been a dear friend and a strong advocate for people with diabetes and their families. Her review provided the additional perspective of a person living successfully with diabetes.

Our families play a major part in our lives. Mike's wife, Gerri, has unselfishly supported our efforts to make our vision a reality. Her contributions go well beyond the sections she wrote for the book and her early reading of the manuscript. Her love and independent commitment to people with diabetes have been an inspiration. She truly has weathered the many storms of Mike's diabetes. Marti's late husband, Jim, provided his love and support for her work for many years and his spirit lingers. We love you both. Our children, Melissa and Michael, Douglas and Alexandra, and Adrian have provided additional motivation and much joy. Hopefully, their world will be enriched by our work. Our mothers and other family members encouraged us to pursue our vision. In particular, Marti's sister, Marilyn Hollingsworth, was an early reader who provided the perspective of one who lived with chronic illness for many years.

We would be seriously remiss if we did not mention the volunteers and staff of the American Diabetes Asociation, and particularly John Graham, who inspired us. Our dear friends, Bunny and Bob Reed, have been unswerving with their cheers and encouragement.

We are also grateful to Jon Anderson and our other friends at Running Press who understood our vision from the onset and helped make this book possible. Our editor, Deborah Grandinetti, truly showed us the way.

Introduction

You may be thinking "Not another diabetes book. There are already hundreds of them, and I barely have time to read one, much less read them all." We agree. However, we believe this is the one that you really have to read. *The Little Diabetes Book You Need to Read* is truly the most important because it prepares you for *living* with diabetes. Most of the other books focus just on *treating* diabetes. This book focuses on *you*, rather than diabetes alone. It recognizes that *you and only you* have the *power* to manage your diabetes. We can't stress that enough.

The power of choice is in your hands. We will explain how to work with your health care providers to build a treatment and self-management plan that capitalizes on *your* strengths, and suits *your* lifestyle. There are a number of different options for managing diabetes, which we will address thoroughly later in the book. We will also give you a step-by-step process to help you make the best choices from your menu of options. This process will empower you to manage diabetes on your own terms, in the way that works best for you. **Successful self-management requires that you adapt diabetes to fit your life instead of adapting your life to diabetes.**

Realize that it is not necessary, nor is it in your best interest, to follow a one-size-fits-all regimen for diabetes. The changes people struggle with most in their lives are those that feel imposed rather than chosen. It is human nature to resist making changes other people tell us to make. You will do far better with a treatment plan that you have played a major part in designing yourself. You are more likely to reduce your risk for complications if you do. As you know, diabetes can lead to some very serious and sometimes fatal physical complications such as heart attacks, strokes, kidney failure, and blindness. The best way to prevent or delay these, as two landmark research studies have shown, is to keep your blood sugar close to normal levels. That's no easy task for anyone with diabetes. Creating a diabetes management plan that works for you will put you far ahead of the game.

In addition, the very process of creating your own treatment plan will give you a framework for making the many decisions you face every day. Having a framework to guide you may help you feel more in control and less overwhelmed. The goal is not to change you, but to help you choose and make the changes *you* want.

That is why we believe this book should be the starting point for your diabetes care. *The Little Diabetes Book You Need to Read* is essential reading whether you are newly diagnosed, or have lived with diabetes for years. It applies no matter what type of diabetes you have, including pre-diabetes. It is also helpful if you have a loved one with diabetes and want to better understand your role in providing support. In fact, we've created special sections just for you under the heading, "A Special Message for Family and Friends."

ABOUT THE AUTHORS

We have the experience to guide you in this area because we have spent decades learning about diabetes and helping others live with it. We don't pretend to have all the answers, but we do have a good handle on the questions you're likely to have and the day-to-day issues you face.

Martha (Marti) has been a diabetes educator since 1983. Marti and her University of Michigan colleague, Bob Anderson, pioneered the once controversial and now widely accepted empowerment approach to diabetes education and treatment. This approach recognizes that behavioral changes, which are so essential to effective diabetes care, will only occur when patients understand and choose the specific changes they wish to make.

Michael (Mike) developed his expertise by living with diabetes for more than 23 years and suffering a number of its serious complications. Much of Mike's understanding is based on personal experience and self-study.

In 2002-2003, we served together as Chair of the Board (Mike) and President, Health

Care & Education (Marti), of the American Diabetes Association. We have spent years speaking with thousands of people with diabetes and their family members. From those encounters, some common themes emerged. One is that people with diabetes are much more likely to be struggling with how to live with diabetes than with the medical aspects of treatment. That was true for Mike as well. In fact, the seeds for this book were planted when Mike confided that he had not been very well prepared to manage his diabetes at the time he was diagnosed. Marti asked what it would have taken to be better prepared. That conversation led to the realization of how useful this kind of book could be.

HOW THIS BOOK IS ORGANIZED

The Little Diabetes Book You Need to Read is grounded in the empowerment approach Marti and her colleague, Bob Anderson, pioneered. Empowerment is discovering the strength that already exists within you, so you can successfully take charge of your diabetes and your life. Finding this strength is a process that requires you to learn, to "do" and to keep doing. Therefore, this book is divided into three main sections.

The "Learning" section has three chapters. The first focuses on the fundamentals of diabetes as a disease. The second chapter explains how to select and work with the right health care professionals for you, and to get the support you need from them and others. The third helps you better understand your own wants, needs, and capabilities as they relate to diabetes management. The better you understand yourself, the easier it is to incorporate diabetes into your life. Gathering this information will give you the foundation for your self-management plan.

The "Doing" section has three chapters. The first two chapters explain how to build your plan, using guiding principles based on your own preferences, and the strategies likely to work best for you. The third chapter explains how to incorporate these changes into your life to accomplish your goals.

The "What Now?" section, which concludes the book, offers tips on how to stay motivated. It also offers a brief summary of the latest research efforts.

We have two key pieces of advice: First, never forget that *you and only you* have the right and the power to determine how you will live with and manage your diabetes. Second, read this book before you read any of the others, and read it again and again as you continue along your journey with diabetes.

CHAPTER 1:

Who's in Charge? You!

A diagnosis of diabetes is life-changing. This chronic, unrelenting condition requires attention 24 hours a day, seven days a week. It is always present. Almost everything you eat and do—every minute, every hour, every day—affects your diabetes. The 24/7 intensity is part of what makes diabetes so different from most other diseases.

Yet most people who have diabetes spend no more than an hour or two a year with their health care professionals. Who will manage it for the remaining 8,758 hours if not you? That is why the primary responsibility rests with you and not your health care professionals.

While there are effective medications and therapies for managing diabetes, there is no cure. Your doctor can't take away the burden, nor tell you what to do each time you need to make a decision about what and how much to eat, what physical activity to pursue, or how much medicine to take, especially if you are using insulin. Similarly, no one else can make you lose weight or become more physically active, two strategies that can help you feel better today and reduce your risk of developing the serious complications of diabetes; nor can anyone else make you take your medicines. When it comes down to it, you must manage diabetes *for yourself.* After all, you are the one who reaps the benefits or suffers the negative effects of your decisions.

The sooner you realize that you and only you have the power to manage your diabetes, the better off you are. That was Mike's experience:

— *Mike Speaks* —

When I was diagnosed with diabetes over 23 years ago, diabetes educators were not nearly as available as they are today. In fact, when a dietitian came to meet me during my initial hospitalization, my doctor told me to just "humor" her! As a result, much of my understanding about diabetes was self-taught from whatever reading materials I managed to find (without, I might add, the convenience of the internet!). So, it was a very slow learning process that dealt mostly with science and biology—the pancreatic mechanics. At the beginning, I was ordered to take a daily shot of insulin and follow a strict diet made up of complicated food exchanges that I still to this day do not fully understand.

This did not work for me at all. I finally figured out that diabetes is a largely self-managed disease, and I was the "self." While my health care providers were available to guide me in the many decisions that I faced on a daily basis, the choices always remained mine. I was forced to figure out for myself how to take charge of my diabetes. I learned through trial and error—mostly error. Not until much later did I learn that I could develop my own care plan that fit better with my lifestyle needs and career demands. And my results improved dramatically.

That is not to suggest that it has been easy. I struggle to keep my blood sugar levels within my target range, and many days I feel like I should have done more. While my anger about having diabetes has decreased significantly, I still have fears about my future and am often frustrated when my best efforts fall short. Despite these feelings, however, I now understand that the responsibility for managing my diabetes is mine alone. While perfection is not attainable, I have learned that through diligent efforts I can significantly improve my outcomes. If only someone had explained my role to me sooner, I might have been able to avoid some of the early anger and frustration and maybe even some of the other complications that I have experienced.

— *Marti Speaks* —

My journey with diabetes is different from Mike's since it is based on my professional, not personal, experiences. Although I am a nurse and a diabetes educator, my patients have always taught me much more than I have ever taught them. At the time when Mike was diagnosed, the approach to people with diabetes was largely as he described. Health professionals spent a lot of effort trying to get them to do what they thought patients should do based on what they knew about diabetes. In other words, managing the illness was expected to control the patient's life. But now we know that diabetes requires a different approach.

An important lesson I learned through my observations of people with diabetes was that those who took charge of their illness did better, both emotionally and physically. I also learned that when I focused on the personal needs of each patient, my efforts were more effective than when I focused on what

I thought that person needed. About 16 years ago, my colleague Bob Anderson and I used our experiences and observations to define a new approach to diabetes care and education. We called it empowerment. This approach enables people with diabetes to create their own treatment plans, and use them to take charge of their condition. Since that time, Bob and I, along with others, have tested this approach in a variety of research studies among people from diverse backgrounds and situations. And it works. ■

There is more to diabetes than just taking medicines. During the course of a single day, you make hundreds of decisions, consciously or otherwise, that affect your blood sugar level. These decisions influence how you feel physically that day, and may affect your emotional state of mind and future health. Managing diabetes is not about compliance with a treatment regimen that has been designed for you by others. Instead, it is about creating your own plan based on an overall strategy and making choices and changes as you implement it.

Managing diabetes effectively requires that you:

- Learn about the impact and consequences of various choices so you can make informed decisions that keep your blood sugar level (and perhaps other measures like blood pressure) on target.
- Make choices that are based on an understanding of your needs and preferences.
- Evaluate your choices, and make adjustments.

This may seem overwhelming. It can be especially difficult if you try to make these choices without an overall plan to guide you.

That is why it is so important to create and implement a workable plan. In some ways, the process of creating your diabetes plan is similar to building a house. Before you begin, you need to know what you want and what is realistic for you. You then need to work with an architect and other experts, while keeping an eye on the end result. Without a plan, you may end up building a lot of rooms, but probably not your dream house. The most satisfying designs are those that are created by working collaboratively. The same is true when it comes to creating a diabetes self-management plan.

Think of your health care providers as architects. The architect knows how to design a structurally sound building based on his or her educational background and experience, but you are the one who knows what floor plan will work best for the way you live and which styles you like most.

Your plan needs to combine what you know about yourself with what your health care professionals know about diabetes. Medications, meal planning, exercise and monitoring are all part of the plan. So are managing stress, dealing with the emotional side of diabetes, learning how to make changes, and balancing the demands of your illness with other priorities, like family and career. Without a plan, you are more likely to feel as if diabetes is controlling you, rather than the other way around.

A Special Message for Family and Friends

A diagnosis of diabetes is usually overwhelming—not only for the person who has it, but for their family members and friends. Unlike most other illnesses, diabetes is a condition where the major responsibility for its management rests with the person who has it. This requires knowledge, skills, and commitment.

As your family member or friend lives with his or her diabetes, in many ways so will you. The reality is that caring for it can be frustrating and disappointing since self-management efforts do not always yield the expected results. At these times, your support and understanding are critical. This book will help you to develop a better appreciation for what it is like to live with diabetes. It will also help you find the strength and support that you need as well.

A NEW BEGINNING

In the next chapter, we will introduce Four LIFE Steps for Living with Diabetes, a dynamic process that will help you develop the best care plan for you. Consider it a starting point on your journey with diabetes. We want to help you to get on and stay on the right path and avoid some of the common pitfalls. This process combines what Mike has learned through his personal experiences and what Marti has learned from working with many people with diabetes. It will help you to fit all the other information about diabetes you receive into the framework of your own life.

CHAPTER 2:
Four LIFE Steps
for Living with Diabetes

D o you remember when diabetes became real for you? Most people do. For some, that moment was when they first heard, "You have diabetes" or "You have pre-diabetes." For others, it happened gradually over the course of several years. And for still others, developing a complication made it real to them for the first time. Even if your experience is through a close family member or friend, you probably remember the moment when diabetes became something real in your life.

— Mike Speaks —

Soon after I started taking insulin, my body suddenly resumed making insulin on its own. Although I later learned that this "honeymoon" often occurs for a short period of time after diagnosis among people with type 1 diabetes, I was absolutely convinced either that my physician had erred in his initial diagnosis, or that somehow I was miraculously cured. My so-called "honeymoon" soon came to an abrupt end, and, with tears in my eyes, diabetes became very real for me. ■

Real diabetes is not the same as "textbook" diabetes. A textbook is likely to cover clinical concerns (like hypoglycemia and insulin resistance), treatments (like diet and insulin) and measurements (like blood sugar and blood pressure levels). While this information is an essential part of its definition, it is far from the whole story.

Real diabetes is different for everyone. It is something you have to define for yourself based on your own experience with it. Your definition is likely to change over time based on the physical and emotional challenges you face.

— Marti Speaks —

When I was a nursing student, I was assigned to develop a teaching plan for a man who had lived with type 1 diabetes for some time. I spent a great deal of time planning and preparing for this session, and was quite pleased with how it went. After my presentation, he said that while I had done a good job, he was not going to do anything differently in caring for his diabetes. Stunned, I asked him why. He told me that what he was doing was working just fine for him. His statement taught me that he was the one in charge and that he knew what was best for his life. That was my first lesson in the difference between textbook diabetes and real diabetes. ■

THE FOUR *LIFE* STEPS

There is no one way that works for everyone. So why accept someone else's recommendations without question? The four LIFE steps will provide the basis for working with your health care team to create *your* plan. We'll summarize the process here, and return to it in depth in Section II of the book. Although this may seem like a lot of extra work, it will in fact make it easier for you on a day-to-day basis.

We like to think of these as the four LIFE steps for living with your diabetes:

Step 1: Learn all you can about diabetes and yourself

Step 2: Identify your three guiding principles: Role, Flexibility, and Targets

Step 3: Formulate your self-management plan

Step 4: Experiment with and Evaluate your plan

An overview of each step follows. Each step will be discussed in more detail later in the book.

Step 1: Learn All You Can About Diabetes and Yourself

This is the "why" of your plan. Diabetes education is absolutely critical, but it needs to occur at two levels. While it is important to learn all you can about diabetes and how to care for it, it is equally important to understand yourself: your feelings, wants, needs, and capabilities.

A good place to start learning is a diabetes education program in your community. You will also find valuable information in magazines, books and on the internet, and of course, from your health care team. Bt don't take eerything you read at face value. While it can teach you about diabetes in general, only you will know how diabetes affects you.

You need to stay in tune with your body and pay attention to how it responds to medications, the food you eat and the exercise you do, and even your emotions and stress level. Again, what works for one person may or may not work for you.

Also take the time to honestly assess yourself: your feelings, wants, needs and capabilities. What's getting in the way of your efforts to take care of yourself? Is it easy for you to make the time to exercise? Is it hard for you to say "no" to particular foods? Can you afford the foods you want and the medicines you need? These concerns will play a part in shaping your plan. Caring for your diabetes cannot be separated from who you are and how you live your life. You do not live in a laboratory or even a world that always supports your efforts to care for yourself. Your plan needs to consider how you will deal with challenges to your best efforts.

Step 2: Identify Your Guiding Principles: Role, Flexibility, and Targets

Now it is time to begin making some decisions. There are three fundamental principles involved in shaping a plan. The three are:

1. **Your Role.** What role do you want to assume in the design of your plan? Do you want your health care providers to do most of this for you, or do you want to play the lead role and use them more as consultants?
2. **Flexibility.** How much flexibility do you want? Are you willing to take additional

blood sugar readings or give yourself more injections in exchange for additional flexibility?

3. **Targets.** What targets are you trying to hit? For your blood sugar level? Weight? Blood pressure? Cholesterol level?

These three questions address the "what" in your self-management plan. Let's look more closely at each of them.

YOUR ROLE

There is no doubt you are in charge of your diabetes care. You cannot delegate this responsibility to anyone else, no matter how much you may wish to do so. Being in charge is one thing, but *taking* charge is another. Being in charge is inescapable; taking charge is a matter of choice.

Taking charge means that you call the shots, make the decisions, and create your own plan in collaboration with your health care team. Just as in building a house, you can choose a standard design or create your own plan. If you decide that you do not feel ready or willing to take charge of your diabetes, and you want your health care professionals to make a plan for you, you need to tell them. This means that you agree to follow their directions. This does not diminish your responsibility; it simply means you have given the right to make certain decisions to someone else.

This is not an "all or nothing" proposition. Nor is it a final decision. As you live with this condition, it is probable that you will assume more and more of this responsibility for yourself. Initially, for example, you might want your provider to prescribe your treatment, but you may want to be in charge of designing your meal plan. As you learn more about how your body responds to the different therapies, you may want to become more involved in the decision process, and consider the positives and negatives of the various options that you can pursue.

On the other hand, if you know that you are the kind of person who likes to make decisions and take action in other situations, you may feel ready to take charge of your diabetes from the very beginning. Or you may gradually assume this responsibility.

There is no one right way, just the way that will work best for you. As you take on this role, your relationship with your healthcare professionals will change as well. You will each have different roles to play as you become collaborators and partners.

FLEXIBILITY

Once that decision is made, consider how much flexibility you want and need in your life. Some people find it easier to follow a strict meal plan and timetable. Others want the ability to change their daily routines to suit their own schedules.

One thing to keep in mind is that more flexibility often means more work. In order to have more flexibility, you may need to make more daily decisions and monitor your blood sugar more often or take more injections. That is the trade-off.

CHOOSING YOUR TARGETS

Choosing your targets comes next. What targets will you select for your blood sugar, weight, blood pressure and cholesterol levels? Ask your health care professionals for advice, and be sure to let them know the targets you have chosen and why. Most of the daily decisions you make in diabetes care are designed to help you reach those targets. It is hard to make choices without a goal in mind. But remember that these are targets and not absolutes.

Setting blood sugar, weight, and other targets can be tricky. While everyone would like to meet the goals recommended by experts, it may not be practical depending on where you start. It may make more sense to establish an easier-to-accomplish intermediate goal as you strive toward your ultimate targets.

Step 3: Formulate Your Self-Management Plan

Now you are ready to formulate your plan. This is the "how" of self-management. In Chapter 7, we'll detail the many options available to you, which include meal planning, exercise, medications, insulin, blood sugar monitoring, stress management, and emotional support. We will show you how to shape those strategies around your preferences and needs. This is how you create the plan you can use day by day.

Step 4: Experiment with and Evaluate Your Plan

This is the "doing" part of your self-management plan. Turning your plan into action involves making choices and often making changes. Making changes is really just the natural culmination of the choices you make to implement your LIFE plan. When you focus on the change, rather than on the daily choices, it becomes daunting. If the choices are consistent with a clear-cut overall objective, the decision about what changes you want to make will follow as a natural consequence.

After you formulate the plan and put it into action, you'll want to evaluate what is and what's not working for you. Maybe your plan to reduce your weight by cutting back on your portions is going well, but you want to make more time to exercise. Or perhaps you want to check your blood sugar more often. It's natural to find you need to make adjustments. Diabetes self-management is often a process of trial and error—you try something, evaluate the outcome, and then use that information to guide your choices the next time around.

And, as Mike said earlier, he learned "through trial and error, mostly error." As you evaluate your "experiments," don't worry about the ones that didn't work. Instead, try something else. As you go along, you will no doubt learn more about yourself and your diabetes. The process of making changes is a continuous cycle of choosing, trying, and evaluating the results. Evaluating your experiment goes beyond deciding whether you succeeded or failed. The focus is on what you learn from your efforts.

Making the lifestyle changes you build into your plan may present challenges. Although a few people find this easy, for most of us it is a daily struggle. If that's the case for you, keep yourself motivated by focusing on your choices rather than the ultimate change. By definition, repetitive choices will result in change. In addition, you have control over your daily choices while other factors can affect the end result. It will also be easier if you break the change down into manageable steps.

It's common for people with diabetes to attempt many changes in their life when they are first diagnosed. That's often the first recommendations made by their health care providers. However, the changes tend to be short-lived. People may slide back to their old eating habits or let their exercise program fall to the wayside. Why does this happen? It could be that the individuals initiating those changes never thought through whether they really wanted to make these changes, and if so, why or how. Or it could be they were trying to do too much at once, or did so as an initial response to a frightening diagnosis. Maybe they did so to please their families or health professionals, or maybe, they attempted to make the changes without first putting together a workable plan.

There are two things to keep in mind. First, it is much easier to make changes and stick with them if they are important to you. Again, the changes people struggle with most in their lives are those that feel *imposed* rather than *chosen*. It is human nature to resist making changes others tell us we need to or should make, no matter how well-intentioned their advice.

Second, it is easier to make changes when you believe you will be successful. If you are like most adults, you have probably tried to make changes in your eating or exercise habits at some point in your life. Your per-

— Marti Speaks —

Something I often hear, especially from people who are newly diagnosed, is that they are so overwhelmed by all there is to do that they are unable to do anything. Being told that you have a serious illness and need to lose weight, stop smoking, exercise, check your blood sugar and learn to manage stress is just too much to take in. In these situations, I usually point out that no one expects them to do everything at once. Helping people identify what is most important or of greatest concern gives us a starting point. The same is true for making changes. After all, you have to learn to crawl before you can walk! ■

ception of the success of those experiences will no doubt affect how you feel about your ability to make similar changes to manage your diabetes. While it is important to learn about yourself from those past experiences, try not to let them undermine your self-confidence. Remember, whether you believe you can or cannot, you are probably correct.

STAY THE COURSE

Sticking with your plan is harder than creating it. So how do you stay motivated?

One way is to get support from other people. Your family and friends can be your biggest cheerleaders. But remember that they cannot manage your diabetes for you. That responsibility is yours alone. Be sure to let your family and friends know how they can help and what you need and expect from them. Tell them what they can expect from you in return. They will be better able to understand and support your daily choices if they know what your plan is. Communication is critical and needs to work both ways to avoid conflicts.

Your health care professionals can also provide a great deal of support. Many communities have support groups for people with diabetes and their families. As you evaluate what is available, look for people who are good listeners and who can be a positive influence.

It's Hard Work

We are not suggesting that any of this is easy. After all, you did not volunteer to have diabetes or pre-diabetes. Developing a workable plan requires an understanding of the disease and its effects. It is equally important that you understand yourself—your feelings, wants, needs, and capabilities—and the consequences of your choices. You can learn to take on this responsibility, one step at a time. As you read further, you will learn how to apply clinical information to your diabetes and your life. You will also learn ways to make choices and changes, and how to develop and apply skills and strategies to the barriers you may face. We'll also teach you how to evaluate the positives and negatives of those decisions. Most importantly, you will learn what real diabetes means to you.

A Special Message for Family and Friends

Real diabetes (as opposed to textbook diabetes) will have special meaning for you, just as it does for your loved one with diabetes. We know from research that people who take an active role in their diabetes care do better than people who do not. In addition, people who have the support of their family and friends also do better. You can be most helpful when you know and understand the plan that has been developed. You may even be asked by your loved one to participate in its creation. When your self-management expectations match, it will be easier for you to support each other along your diabetes journey. ■

Part I: Learning

CHAPTER 3:
Know Your Opponent

Just as a good quarterback would never take to the field without first learning all he can about the opposing team, you need to understand all you can about your diabetes. To be sure, diabetes is a worthy opponent. It is normal to feel scared and overwhelmed when you are first diagnosed. Diabetes is a complicated disease. Volumes have been written about it, and more is being discovered every day. We encourage you to learn as much as you can. To get you started, we'll cover the essentials you need to create your self-management plan. This knowledge will put you in a better position to make informed choices and changes in your life.

DIABETES: A TOUGH DISEASE

Make no mistake: diabetes is a tough disease—whether it's type 1 or type 2, gestational or pre-diabetes. Although no illness is pleasant, diabetes is particularly demanding on the people who have it, and those closest to them. As we've said before, the complications are serious, and can be life threatening. Your future health is at stake.

So what exactly is diabetes? Simply stated, it's a condition where there is too much **glucose,**[*] or sugar, trapped in your bloodstream. As a result, the cells in your body are not getting the sugar they need for energy. Without energy, the cells cannot function as they should. Over time, complications can occur.

You may have heard diabetes referred to as "sugar diabetes." That is because many people think of it as a sugar problem. In fact, diabetes is an **insulin** problem. Insulin is the hormone needed to move sugar from the bloodstream into the cells. When you have

---

[*]Words in bold are defined in the Glossary of Terms that starts on page 245. While glucose and sugar are technically not the same thing, they will be used interchangeably throughout this book. It is likely that your health care professionals will use these words interchangeably as well.

diabetes, sugar becomes trapped in your bloodstream because your body does not make enough or any insulin, or cannot effectively use the insulin it does make.

TYPES OF DIABETES

One form of diabetes is called type 1 diabetes. Type 1 diabetes, which used to be called "juvenile" diabetes, is believed to be an autoimmune disease. For reasons no one completely understands, the body's immune system destroys the beta cells of the pancreas. As a result, these cells stop producing insulin. Only about 5 to 10 percent of people with diabetes have type 1. Although type 1 diabetes usually is diagnosed in children and young adults, it is not uncommon for it to develop in adults.

Chances are you have type 2 diabetes, since 90 to 95 percent of people with diabetes have type 2. While it most often occurs in adults, it is becoming more and more common in younger people, and even children. Type 2 diabetes appears to result largely from heredity combined with other factors, such as body weight and lack of physical activity. If you have type 2 diabetes, your pancreas still produces some insulin. As you get older, heavier and less active, however, your cells become more and more resistant to it. Initially, your pancreas is able to make enough insulin to compensate, but as time goes by, the pancreas is just not able to keep up. This is why people with type 2 diabetes often need to take insulin. However, this does not mean that they have developed type 1 diabetes.

Because type 2 diabetes does not present any severe symptoms in the beginning, approximately a third of the people with type 2 diabetes do not even know they have the disease. While it may seem like a good thing to put off knowing that you have a serious disease as long as possible, it's not, because during this time high blood sugar levels are taking a toll on your body. As a result, sometimes type 2 diabetes is not diagnosed until a complication develops. Sadly, that complication might have been prevented with earlier diagnosis and treatment.

Some people mistakenly believe that type 1 diabetes is more serious because people with type 1 need to give themselves shots from the start. However, whether you have type 1 or type 2 , the long-term effects can be the same. Even people with pre-diabetes are at risk for complications. All types of diabetes need to be taken seriously.

A third type is called gestational diabetes. This type develops during pregnancy because the hormones that the placenta normally produces cause the mother to become insulin resistant. If a woman is not able to make enough insulin to overcome the resistance, gestational diabetes develops. Gestational diabetes often goes away after childbirth, but women who experience it are more likely to develop diabetes in future pregnancies and to have type 2 diabetes as they get older.

Finally, there is pre-diabetes, which is also called **impaired glucose tolerance**, or IGT. This means that your blood sugar levels are higher than normal but not high enough for you to be diagnosed with diabetes. It is now estimated that more than 54 million Americans have pre-diabetes and are at high risk for developing type 2 during their life-times. Some people used to call this "border-line" diabetes or a "touch of sugar." They were incorrect. You either have diabetes or pre-diabetes, or you do not. If you are not sure which type of diabetes you have or whether you even have it, ask your health care team. There are simple blood tests that can be done to answer this question. The more you know about what is happening to your body, the better equipped you will be to make informed decisions.

COMPLICATIONS

Diabetes can affect you in many different ways, both physically and emotionally. In the short term, if you have too much sugar in your bloodstream (a condition called

hyperglycemia), you may experience tiredness, irritability, hunger, weight loss, dry
mouth and skin, thirst, increased urination,
and blurred vision. It makes sense that you
feel this way; with the sugar trapped in your
bloodstream, your cells are literally starving
for energy. As your body attempts to get rid
of this extra sugar through more frequent
urination, your thirst increases and you can

— *Marti Speaks* —

*Many people with diabetes tell me that they
feel just fine when their blood sugar is high,
and feel worse once their blood sugar starts to
come down into the target range. It is true that
your body tends to get used to the high levels
of sugar and you may feel as though you are
too low as you start to come into the target
range. But we know from research studies (and
from what Mike and many others have told
me) that once the body adapts to glucose levels in the target range, they have more energy,
are less depressed, and have more "zest for living" than when their levels are high.* ■

become dehydrated. Bringing your blood sugar levels down decreases these effects. You will likely have more energy and feel better both physically and emotionally.

If you have type 1 diabetes and your blood sugar levels remain very high for a period of time, you may experience **ketosis**, which requires immediate medical attention. Ketosis, if left untreated, can lead to **ketoacidosis**, and ultimately to a coma or death. Ketoacidosis commonly occurs at the time a person is first diagnosed with type 1 diabetes. It can also occur after diagnosis during an acute illness, such as an infection or the flu. Developing a plan with your health care team for when you are sick or unable to eat can help you prevent ketoacidosis from occurring or progressing.

Now comes the scariest part. If you have known people with diabetes, you may have seen them develop one or more of its long-term complications. One of the most difficult things about living with diabetes is thinking about the possibility that you may develop these same complications. Over the long term, the effects of diabetes can lead to serious problems and even death. As the sugar flows through the larger blood vessels in your heart, neck, and legs, it can damage the cells in the lining of the blood vessels, causing them to become stiff. This allows plaque to build up in those vessels, which can ultimately result in a heart attack, stroke, or amputation.

High blood sugar levels can also damage the smaller blood vessels in the eyes, causing serious eye disease (called **retinopathy**) or even blindness. Or they may damage the smaller blood vessels in the kidney, leading to kidney disease (called **nephropathy**) and possibly end-stage renal disease. High blood sugar levels can also cause sexual problems, such as **Erectile Dysfunction** (ED) or impotence in men, or difficulty becoming aroused or having an orgasm in women. This is often a great source of frustration, and may lead to depression.

Partners of men who experience ED often find that it makes a big difference in their lives as well. One of the things they often say is that their partners are depressed, angry, or sometimes hesitant to kiss them or show other signs of affection. They often claim to

— *Mike Speaks* —

While the seriousness of cardiovascular disease, blindness, and kidney failure cannot be denied, one complication of high blood sugar levels that men with diabetes often raise privately (but seldom in public) is erectile dysfunction. It is estimated that ED affects up to half of the men who have diabetes. Sadly, many of these men admit that they are too embarrassed to discuss this problem with their health care professionals. Many diabetes publications also avoid the subject, which just adds to the discomfort. Luckily, there are numerous treatments available today that can help. If ED (or the fear of developing ED) is a problem for you, be sure to discuss it with your health care provider. Your silence can only aggravate the problem. ■

miss that intimacy more than they miss sex.

High blood sugar levels can also cause damage to the nerves (called **neuropathy**) resulting in pain or numbness in the legs and feet. When your legs and feet are numb, you

— *Marti Speaks* —

Men are not alone in their concern about sexual functioning. Women with diabetes also talk about how it has affected their sex lives. A common statement is, "I am just too tired." They tell me that by the time they do everything at work and at home that they need to do, and take care of their diabetes, they just want to go to sleep at night. Women with diabetes are also prone to infections that make sex uncomfortable or cause them to feel less desirable. They may experience dryness or respond less easily. How women respond to sex is often related to how they feel about themselves or their partner. Take time to help yourself feel sexy and desirable. Set aside some time with your partner and make it a priority in your lives together. ■

might not realize you have a minor injury until it becomes infected. When the circulation is poor, injuries and infections heal slowly, and could ultimately require an amputation if not treated promptly. For this reason, it is important that you and your provider each check your feet routinely. It is a good idea to take off your shoes and socks automatically at the beginning of each office visit as a reminder to check your feet.

Now for the good news: One of the most important advances in diabetes is the growing understanding of how to treat or prevent its long-term complications. There are effective treatments available.

Two landmark research studies have been conducted, one among people with type 1 diabetes (Diabetes Control and Complications Trial or **DCCT**) and the other among people with type 2 diabetes (United Kingdom Prospective Diabetes Study or **UKPDS**). These studies proved that you can avoid or delay many of the long-term complications by keeping your blood sugar levels closer to recommended levels. In addition, there are better medications and treatments for complications today than in the past. Be sure to remind your health care team to do the necessary tests for these complications so that they can be diagnosed while treatment is most effective.

Another significant, yet rarely discussed, effect of diabetes is its impact on emotional health. A major international research study called DAWN (Diabetes Attitudes Wishes and Needs) found that a significant number of people with diabetes experience anxiety, distress, depression, and other difficult emotions. It is not unusual to feel guilty about getting diabetes, or angry about having the responsibility for managing it thrust upon you. Or, you may feel frustrated that you can't achieve the blood sugar targets you have set for yourself despite what you feel are great personal sacrifices. Perhaps you fear the long-term complications that can occur over time. Depression is common among people with diabetes, and many people report feeling hostile, anxious and stressed out. These negative emotions can make it harder for you to care for your diabetes, which, in turn, can add to your feelings of anger, guilt, hostility, anxiety, and depression.

WHAT YOU CAN DO

There have been enormous strides in the treatment of diabetes over the past twenty years. Rest assured that with newer drugs and devices, and the continually increasing understanding of the disease and availability of education, your diabetes is more manageable today than it ever has been.

Experts recommend target ranges for a fasting or pre-meal blood sugar level of 90 (5.0 mmol/l) to 130 mg/dl (7.2 mmol/l), and below 180 mg/dl (10 mmol/l) one to two hours after a meal. These recommendations from the American Diabetes Association are based on the research studies described above and will give you the best chance to prevent complications. You and your health care team may choose to set your personal targets at different levels. The important thing is to choose a target so that both you and your health care team are clear about your goals.

There are a number of good ways to manage diabetes and pre-diabetes. Since diabetes is a condition where there is too much sugar in your bloodstream, you might think, why not just stop eating anything that contains sugar? If only it were that simple! First, many of the products that you buy in grocery stores contain sugar as an ingredient. It is not just limited to candies, cookies, and other sweets. That is why it is so important to read the nutrition labels on packaged foods. Secondly, almost all of the **carbohydrates** you eat break down into glucose as they are digested. Carbohydrates include bread, pasta, rice and other starches, fruits and vegetables, as well as sugar. Your body needs carbohydrates as a source of energy. Remember that the problem in diabetes is not sugar, but a lack of insulin. So even if you stopped eating sugar, your blood sugar level would probably not always stay in the normal range.

Before you got diabetes, your body kept your blood sugar levels within the normal range by making some insulin all the time (**basal level**) and producing a burst, or **bolus**, of insulin when your blood sugar started to rise. Between meals and overnight, your liver released glucose it stored throughout the day. The pancreas made just enough insulin so that this glucose went into the cells and gave you enough energy for your body to function during these times. When you ate, your pancreas made an additional bolus of insulin to keep the blood sugar level in the normal range. The amount of the bolus insulin your pancreas produced was roughly proportional to the amount of carbohydrate in the meal.

Now that you have diabetes, this no longer occurs. Therapies for diabetes are designed to mimic the function of the pancreas as closely as possible. Because your body is not producing enough insulin to keep up with the demand, all of the treatments are designed to give you the insulin you need or to help you use it more effectively.

The treatment for type 1 diabetes is pretty straightforward. People with this kind of diabetes must take insulin from the time of diagnosis—because their bodies make no insulin. The challenge is figuring how much insulin to take and when. The treatment for type 2 diabetes is more complex. Because it is progressive, the treatment will often become more extensive over time, especially as people age, gain weight and become less physically active. As a result, people with type 2 diabetes may start their treatment by making basic lifestyle changes, such as exercising and losing weight, changing their diet, or using a meal plan. Current thinking among experts, however, is that it is best to start taking one of the oral medications, metformin, right away.

Whether you start with a pill or add it later, it is common to add a second or third pill, another injectable medicine, or insulin over time. Sometimes, insulin is prescribed at the start for people who are newly diagnosed with type 2 diabetes if their blood sugar levels are very high. The insulin may be discontinued when these levels reach a more desirable level. Most people with type 2 diabetes will eventually need insulin to keep their blood sugar levels on target, however. Adding new therapies, or changing them, does not mean that you are worse or that you have failed to manage effectively. It is part of the natural progression of diabetes and simply means you need more help to keep your blood sugar levels where you want them.

There is no one best way to treat diabetes. The best treatment is the one that is easiest or most possible for you, helps you reach your goals and blood sugar targets, has the fewest side effects, and is affordable.

— Marti Speaks —

You may have heard type 1 diabetes called insulin-dependent and type 2 diabetes called non-insulin dependent diabetes. It is true that people with type 1 diabetes are dependent on taking insulin to live. However, more and more people with type 2 diabetes are taking insulin to keep their blood sugar on target. This does not mean that they now have type 1 diabetes. It just means that they need to take insulin to manage their blood sugar levels. ■

Insulin

The most well-known and effective "medicine" for treating diabetes is insulin. Unfortunately, insulin cannot be taken as a pill. You can choose, however, from different tools for taking insulin such as syringes, pens, or insulin pumps. If you are concerned about giving yourself shots (and who isn't?), it may help to know that the new, very small needles make giving yourself shots less painful than you might think. In some cases, inhaled insulin can be used instead of injections. You may want to ask your health care professionals whether this is an option for you.

— Mike Speaks —

As with so many things in life, the thought of giving yourself a shot is more frightening than actually doing it. This really came home to me at a recent visit to our local diabetes camp when I watched scores of children "shoot up" together before dinner. A pretty, petite 8-year-old girl was so proud and excited to be giving herself a shot for the very first time as all the onlookers cheered and applauded her courage (and some of the adults struggled not to cry). I am sure that neither she nor I will ever forget that moment. If an 8-year-old can do it, chances are that someone who is older can, too. It just takes a little courage at first. Many people agree with me that injections are less difficult for them than sticking their fingers with a lancet. ■

There are also different types of insulins. Some work very quickly, and are taken to provide a bolus of insulin when you eat a meal. These are either rapid- or fast-acting insulins. They start to work quickly and their effects last anywhere from 2 to 6 hours depending on the specific type and other factors. Others work more gradually and may last up to 24 hours to provide a basal level of insulin. Many people take more than one type, separately or in combination. Once again, the type or types you use will depend on your blood sugar levels and how intensively you want to manage your diabetes. This is a critical subject for you to explore with your health care team. The table on pages 90–91 describes the available types of insulin and their uses.

Although most people still think of insulin as a treatment for type 1 diabetes, insulin is often used by people with type 2 diabetes to manage their blood sugar levels. If you have type 2 diabetes, over time your pancreas will become less and less able to make enough insulin. Needing to take insulin at that point does not mean you are worse off; it just means that your body needs more help to keep your blood sugar where you want it. The bottom line is to keep your blood sugar levels within your target range.

Pills

There are several types of pills for treating type 2 diabetes. Different types work differently, but all help to keep your blood sugar level in the target range. Because the pills do different things, they are often combined to give you the maximum results. For example, you may take one pill to help your pancreas make more insulin, another to help slow down the production of glucose by the liver and another to increase the sensitivity of your cells to insulin. You may also take insulin or other injectable along with these pills. Even if you start with one medication, such as metformin, you may add one or two other pills. Everyone is different, and it often takes some experimentation to find the right combination for you. Don't be discouraged if the first approach is not quite right. Whenever your provider recommends a new medication, ask what it is used for, when to take it in relation to eating, what side effects you might have, how it will interact with your other medicines and, if it's a concern for you, how much it will cost. The different types of pills are described in the table on pages 92–93.

If you take insulin or certain types of pills to treat your diabetes, you need to know about another problem that could arise. If your dose of insulin or some pills is too large, or if you eat later or less than usual, or exercise more than usual, your blood sugar levels could drop to a dangerously low level (a condition called **hypoglycemia** or a "reaction"). A blood sugar level of less than 70 mg/dl (3.9 mmol/l) is usually considered too low. You may feel shaky, sweaty, weak, irritable, and confused. This is a serious situation requiring immediate action to raise your blood sugar level by taking a quick acting source of sugar. When treated, the blood sugar comes back up fairly quickly (within 15 minutes). Left untreated, this can result in a coma or death. If you take insulin or oral medications, ask your health care team to tell you how to prevent, recognize, and treat hypoglycemia.

— Mike Speaks —

Even after all these years, going low is a terrifying experience. I am fortunate enough to still be able to detect when it happens. Nevertheless, when my blood sugar drops suddenly and I begin to feel symptoms, I sometimes panic. Although I know better, my emotional response sometimes leads me to overreact by taking too much sugar, causing my blood sugar to soar. It becomes a vicious cycle with which I and many others still struggle. In these situations, most health care professionals recommend that you follow the so-called "Rule of 15s"—take 15 grams of glucose, wait 15 minutes and retest your blood sugar level; if it is till too low, keep repeating until your target level is reached. During the process, you may feel it is not helping, but give it a chance. Once you feel confident that it does work, it is easier to avoid "bingeing" to treat a low. ■

Other Diabetes Medications

There are two classes of medications that came on the market in 2005. In some ways, they are similar because both mimic hormones (**amylin** and **GLP-1**) the body normally makes. They both help lower your blood sugar levels after meals. They slow down how quickly food is absorbed, so you feel full faster, and slow down the production of glucose by the liver. However, the way each works and for whom they are recommended is different. At the time this book went to press, both drugs were available only as injections. Both have weight loss as a side effect, which many people think is a good thing. Side effects are not always bad! These medications are described in the table.

Other Diabetes Medications			
TYPE	NAME	HOW OFTEN TO TAKE	WHEN
Amylin Incretin mimetic	Symlin (amylin)	2-3 times per day	Before meals
GLP-1 Incretin mimetic	Byetta (exenatide)	2 times per day	Before breakfast and supper

Lifestyle

Certain lifestyle changes—like losing weight, and exercising—have been shown to benefit people who have or are at risk for type 2 diabetes. In fact, a large study called the Diabetes Prevention Program (DPP) concluded that many people who were at high risk for developing type 2 diabetes could delay (or possibly even prevent) its onset by losing weight and exercising. Surprisingly, the weight loss needed was only five to seven percent of body weight. That's 9 to 13 pounds, for instance, for someone who weighs 180 pounds. This study showed that the amount of exercise needed was about 30 minutes of walking five days a week. Although this is not trivial to do, it may be reassuring to know that you do not necessarily have to get down to your high school weight or join a gym. Many people who already have type 2 diabetes notice lower blood sugar levels with this same amount of weight loss and activity.

Although lifestyle is often thought of as part of the treatment for type 2 and pre-diabetes, it is actually beneficial for treating type 1 diabetes as well. Many of the decisions you need to make each day have to do with maintaining the balance between what you eat, your physical activity and your medications. In general, food and stress cause your blood sugar to go up, and physical activity and medicines bring it down. The trick (and it really is a trick!) is to keep your blood sugar at levels that will provide your body with the energy it needs, while not so high as to cause short and long-term problems. Easier said than done! Maintaining this balance can be the most challenging and frustrating thing about caring for diabetes.

If you have type 1, chances are that as you get older you will tend to become heavier and less active, which adds to insulin resistance. You may also gain weight if you manage your diabetes more intensively because insulin helps your body to use food more efficiently. In addition, as your blood sugar level comes down, you will lose less glucose in your urine. Your body now has those calories to use. So even if you eat the same amount you may gain weight. If this is a concern, ask your provider for a referral to a dietitian or certified diabetes educator.

Another lifestyle challenge is managing stress. We all have a great deal of tension in our lives, and caring for diabetes is yet another source of stress. When you feel stressed, your body produces hormones (adrenalin and cortisol) to get you ready to react quickly. These hormones break down glucose your body stores for later use, which in turn generally raise your blood sugar, although some people find that it causes a drop in blood sugar. If you have type 1 diabetes and your blood sugar goes up, you probably do not have enough insulin on board to bring it back down. If you have type 2 diabetes, your blood sugar is likely to remain high, since these stress hormones also increase insulin resistance. Although you cannot eliminate all of the stress in your life, including stress from diabetes, you can learn to recognize and manage it more effectively.

We want to add a final word about stress. Many people believe their diabetes was caused by a stressful event. In fact, stress does not directly cause diabetes, but it can hasten its development among people who were already at risk.

MEASURING YOUR PROGRESS
Monitoring Blood Sugar

As you can see, the treatments for diabetes are designed to help your body function closer to the way it did before you developed it. However, the treatments cannot work without your help. Before you developed diabetes, your body automatically balanced your insulin output with your diet, exercise or lack of it, stress level, etc. Now you have to create that balance yourself. Many of the decisions you make throughout the day are related to balancing all of the factors that affect blood sugar levels—something your

— *Marti Speaks* —

Although we now take them for granted, I remember seeing a home blood glucose meter for the first time in the late 1970s. Before each measurement, you needed to calibrate a rather large, heavy machine that required a big, hanging drop of blood, obtained using a metal lancet. After waiting one or two minutes, you had to rinse just the right amount of blood off the strip and blot it dry. For all of this work, your blood sugar was shown on a dial so that it was hard to figure out the exact reading. When I was first shown this machine by a sales body used to do automatically. It would be easier if your internal gauges told you what your actual sugar levels were so you would know exactly what to do. But they do not. Fortunately, there are blood sugar monitors to give you real-time readings at home so that you have the information you need. You no longer have to go to the doctor's office or

representative, I was very skeptical. In fact, I told him that no one would ever go through this painful process. But I was wrong. People with diabetes wanted this information badly enough that they were willing to endure the pain and inconvenience. Over the years, the technology has evolved, making meters more accurate, user-friendly, and available for almost everyone with diabetes. Most people with diabetes cannot begin to imagine life without their meters. ■

lab to have blood drawn and wait for the results to get accurate readings.

Home blood glucose monitoring is one of the most valuable tools you have for making informed decisions in the treatment of your diabetes. There are a number of different, user-friendly blood glucose monitors on the market today. These devices give quick results and are relatively easy to use. Fortunately, the cost for meters and strips is covered today by most health care plans, including Medicare. Ask your health care providers for help in selecting one that will work well for you and is covered by your insurance or other third-party payment plan. If you are not covered, they may be able to direct you to sources where you can get a meter and supplies at little or no cost.

Like every other tool, a glucose monitor is only as good as the way you use it. When you see a number that is in your target range, do you stop and say "good job" or think about what you did that helped? When you see a number that is too high, do you make adjustments in your medications or other parts of your plan or use it to feel bad about yourself? Do you skip monitoring to avoid "bad news" or do you check more often when you think you are out of your target range so you can take action? Remember that blood sugar readings are not a judgment or a score on a test. Your readings provide you with the ability to make informed choices. Monitoring is for *you*, not just your health care professionals. As you live your life with diabetes, your monitor likely will become your best friend and ally! If you are unclear about what the numbers mean or how to use the information, ask your health care professionals for help.

A reading from your blood glucose meter gives you a snapshot of where your blood sugar level is at a particular moment. There is an equally valuable test called the **A1C** that measures your average blood sugar level over the past 3 to 4 months. It shows you the big picture of how your treatment is working. It also gives you an idea about your risk for the complications. Although this blood test is normally done in a physician's office or laboratory, you can buy a home A1C test at your pharmacy. Insurance coverage varies, so you may want to check with your carrier before purchasing them.

The chart below shows the relationship between A1C values and the incidence of certain complications. As you can see, the higher the A1C, the more you are at risk. Lowering your A1C can have a dramatic effect on your risk.

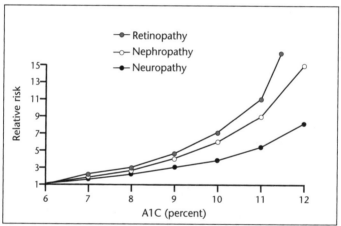

Skyler J: Endocrinology and Metabolism Clinics 1996; 25:243-254.

The American Diabetes Association recommends an A1C level of less than 7 percent, which equates to an average blood sugar reading of approximately 170 mg/dl (9.5 mmol/l). The American Association of Clinical Endocrinologists recommends a level of 6.5 percent which equates to an average blood sugar level of 154 mg/dl (8.6 mmol/l).These recommendations are based on research studies (DCCT, UKPDS) showing the benefits of keeping your blood sugar level close to the normal range, which is 4 to 6 percent. A table that translates A1C levels to average blood sugar levels appears on page 89.

Other Measures

Managing diabetes is about more than just insulin and blood sugar. The UKPDS showed that high blood pressure also increases your risk for the complications of diabetes. In addition, if you have diabetes and high blood pressure, you are two to four times more likely to develop heart disease and five times more likely to have a stroke than people without diabetes. As a result, the American Diabetes Association and the American Heart Association have created recommendations for blood pressure and **cholesterol** levels and timetables for testing them. These recommendations are listed on page 89 and are based on multiple research studies. Many of the lifestyle decisions you make to manage your diabetes will positively affect these values. Lowering your blood sugar level will often lower your **triglycerides**, another type of fat found in the bloodstream. In addition, blood pressure and cholesterol can be regulated by medications. Taking charge of your diabetes means paying attention to these recommendations as well. So ask your health care team about your results, how often you need these tests done and if they would recommend treatment.

— *Mike Speaks* —

Whether it is an A1C, blood pressure or cholesterol check, or even a routine blood sugar reading, it is important to remember that the results are only a tool for evaluating what worked and did not work in the past, so you know what needs to be done going forward. They are in no way a measure of your ability or character. ■

FINANCES

Diabetes can be costly for the person who has it. It has been estimated that the annual cost of having diabetes exceeds $13,000. Most of this cost relates to medications and supplies such as blood glucose monitoring strips. Fortunately, the American Diabetes Association has been successful in its efforts to have legislation adopted in 46 states and the District of Columbia that mandates health insurance coverage of diabetes monitoring supplies and diabetes education. These efforts have helped to reduce the cost for those who are fortunate enough to have health insurance coverage. But the coverage will vary from one insurance company to another. Check with your insurer (including Medicare and Medicaid) to confirm exactly which medicines and supplies (including brands and the number of strips) are covered, and what your co-payments will be. Health insurance companies maintain lists (or **formularies**) of the specific drugs and supplies and the quantities of each for which they will pay, and these lists will vary from one insurer to the next. Some plans may also set different levels of co-pays for medications. This information is also included in the formulary.

Once you have this information, you may want to discuss it with your health care providers to identify the drugs and supplies that will be least costly to you and still provide the desired results. Fortunately, there are numerous options from which to choose. Most pharmaceutical companies have introduced programs to make their products available to people who might not be able to afford them otherwise. Your doctor or pharmacist can provide information about these services. Keep in mind that insurance coverage is likely to change, and some state coverage mandates may be challenged because of continued pressure to reduce healthcare costs.

As you can see, diabetes is complex and there is a lot to know. It is also important to realize that diabetes treatments involve a lot of trial and error. What works for some people, may not work for others, and what worked for you yesterday may not be as effective today or tomorrow. Just be patient as you and your health care professionals work together to design the course that works for you. Remember there is no one "best" way to treat diabetes.

— *Mike Speaks* —

One of the most surprising lessons for me was how individualized diabetes treatment is for each person who has it. Friends of mine sometimes seem to be using plans that are very different, but their plans work for them just as mine does for me. I have come to realize that our bodies all respond differently, and that it is very difficult to predict what will happen. Diabetes management sometimes feels like it is hit or miss. That is why it is so important to keep track of your activities and blood sugar readings so that you can review them with your healthcare team and remove some of the guesswork. ■

This chapter was just a brief (really it is brief given the amount of information that is out there) summary to help you begin to formulate your self-management plan. Know-

THE LITTLE DIABETES BOOK YOU NEED TO READ

ledge is power, so the more you learn, the more empowered you will be. If you want to know more, ask your provider for a referral to a diabetes educator or diabetes education program. Diabetes education is one of the most valuable resources you have at your disposal. The resources listed starting on page 250 may also be of help to you.

A Special Message for Family and Friends

Diabetes is very complicated. The more you know about it, the easier it will be to understand the many peaks and valleys your loved one and you will experience. One way to expand your knowledge beyond reading this book is to attend diabetes education programs available in your community. Many of these programs include ideas and information specifically for family and friends. Discuss with your loved one whether your participation would be helpful. ■

Recommended Monitoring

	TARGET LEVEL	WHEN TO MEASURE
A1C	6.5-7%	Every 3-6 months
Blood Pressure	Less than 130/80	Every routine provider visit
Cholesterol LDL HDL Triglycerides	Less than 100mg/dl More than 40mg/dl Less that 150mg/dl	At least once per year
Urine Albumin (protein)	Less that 30ug/mg	Once per year
Dilated Retinal Examination	Not applicable	Once per year

Average Plasma Sugar Levels Compared to A1C Levels

AIC LEVEL	AVERAGE BLOOD SUGAR	
	Mg/dL	mmol/l
6%	135	7.5
7%	170	9.5
8%	205	11.5
9%	240	13.5
10%	275	15.5
11%	310	17.5
12%	345	19.5

Type of insulin

TYPE	COLOR	EFFECTS
Rapid-acting Lispro Aspart Apidra	Clear	Begins to work in 15 minutes, peaks in about 1 hour, and continues to work for 2.4 hours
Short-acting **Regular** Reli-On	Clear	Begins to work in 30 minutes, peaks in 2-5 hours and continues to work for 6-16 hours
Intermediate-acting NPH Lente	Cloudy	Begins to work in 1-2 hours, peaks 4-12 hours later, and is effective for 12-22 hours
Long-acting **Glargine** Detemir	Clear	Begins to work in 5 hours and lasts 20-24 hours
Mixtures Rapid- or short-acting plus intermediate	Cloudy	Begins to work in 15-30 minutes, lasts about 24 hours
Inhaled Exubera	Powder	Begins to work in 10-20 minutes, lasts about 6 hours

WHEN TO TAKE	WHEN TO TEST BLOOD SUGAR
5-15 minutes before eating	2 hours after that meal.
30 minutes before eating	2 hours after that meal and before the next meal
Before breakfast and/or before dinner or bedtime Before breakfast and before dinner.	Before breakfast and before dinner
Before breakfast or before dinner or half dose at each time.	Before breakfast and at bed-time
Before breakfast and/or before dinner	Before breakfast and before dinner
Less than 10 minutes before meals	2 hours after that meal

Types of Pills

TYPE	NAME
Sulfonylureas Stimulates the pancreas to release more insulin	Glimepiride (Amaryl) Glipizide (Glucotrol, Glucotrol XL) Glyburide (Diabeta, Micronase, Glynase Prestab)
Biguanides Keep the liver from releasing too much glucose	Metformin (glucophage, Glucophage XR) Metformin + a sulfonylurea (Glucovance, Metaglip)
Glitinides Stimulate the pancreas to release more insulin	Repaglinide (Prandin) Nateglinide (Starlix)
Thiazolidinediones Make muscle cells more sensitive to insulin	Rosiglitazone (Avandia) Pioglitazone (Actos) Rosiglitazone + metformin (Avandamet) Pioglitizone + metformin (Actoplus met) Roseiglitizone + glimepiride (Avandaryl)
Alpha-Glucosidase Inhibitors Slow the digestion of starches	Acarbose (precose) Miglitol (glyset)
DPP-IV Inhibitors Stimulate the release of insulin and slows down the release of glucose	Januvia (Sitagliptin) Janumet (sitagliptin+metformin

HOW OFTEN TO TAKE	WHEN TO TAKE
Once a day 1 or 2 times a day	Take glipizide 1/2 hour before meals.
1 or 2 times a day	
1 or 2 times a day	Take with largest meal of the day to decrease stom- ach upset.
1 or 2 times a day	
3-4 times a day 3-4 times a day	Take 1-30 minutes before meals.
1 or 2 times a day	
Once a day 2 times a day	
3-4 times a day	Take with the first bite of each meal.
Once a day	Take daily with or without food

CHAPTER 4:
Know Your Team

Just as an effective quarterback would never consider taking the field without knowing his opponent, he would never consider going into a game without the support of the best possible team. It is not enough just to know the team members; you also have to understand the positions they play, and their different skills and abilities. Your diabetes team includes you, numerous health care professionals, your family, and your friends. Some will play the role of coaches, some players, and some cheerleaders. However, you will always be your team's quarterback who calls and executes the plays.

While the number of people with diabetes in the United States and throughout the world has been growing at a frighteningly fast pace over the past ten years, the number of health care professionals available to treat them has not grown at nearly the same rate. As a result, some experts say that the fastest growing group of primary providers in diabetes is actually the people who have the disease! This is all the more reason why people with diabetes must be active members of their health care teams.

YOUR HEALTH CARE PROVIDERS

Think of your health care providers as your coaches and fellow players. For most of you, your main health care provider will be your primary care practitioner. Your primary care provider may be a family physician, an internist, a nurse practitioner, or a physician's assistant. Although many primary care providers are experts in diabetes, if you want or need a more specialized approach (particularly if you have decided to manage your diabetes intensively), you may also wish to consult with an **endocrinologist**, a physician whose practice is focused on treating diabetes. You can receive all of your care from an endocrinologist, or make occasional visits for a "tune up."

— Marti Speaks —

A common question patents ask is whether they should see a specialist. There is no hard and fast rule. Generally, it is recommended that people with type 1 diabetes receive their diabetes care from someone who specializes in diabetes, such as an endocrinologist or internist who focuses on treating people with diabetes. People with type 2 diabetes may choose to see an endocrinologist either periodically or routinely. If you are being followed by your primary care provider, and your treatment plan appears to be working, then you probably do not need to see a specialist. But if you are not satisfied with your therapy, then a visit to a specialist may be in order. A diabetes specialist may be especially helpful as you begin insulin, you want more intensive therapy, or if you develop a complication. ■

Your main diabetes practitioner will be the one to prescribe your medications and to follow your overall progress, which may include detecting and treating complications. If you or your provider believes that additional expertise is needed, your provider can refer you to other health care specialists.

Diabetes Educators

The diabetes educator is another essential member of your team. Diabetes educators are usually nurses or dietitians who are specially trained to teach people how to manage their disease on a day to day basis. If you are taking insulin, chances are that a diabetes educator will be the one to teach you how to give yourself a shot or how to use your insulin pump or inhaler. If you are using more intensive treatments, they can help you to adjust and regulate your insulin doses. Some specialists have diabetes educators right on staff for easy access.

Diabetes educators can help you with your emotional and psychological concerns as well. They generally can be reached by telephone or email and are often more readily available than your practitioner. Some have undergone rigorous testing to become **Certified Diabetes Educators** or **CDEs.** While most Certified Diabetes Educators are nurses or dietitians, CDEs can also be pharmacists, psychologists, podiatrists or even physicians. You can locate them on the AADE website at www.aadenet.org or the ADA website at www.diabetes.org.

— *Marti Speaks* —

I have been a diabetes educator for more than twenty years. My role is to help people learn about diabetes so they can make informed decisions. I always tell people I have the best job in the world – I get to bring help and hope to those with diabetes. There is nothing more rewarding than to see the look on the face of someone who truly "gets it" for the first time and to feel their sense of accomplishment and confidence. Sadly, only about 30 percent of patients receive formal diabetes education. Often, the provider forgets to make the referral or ask if one is wanted. Ask your provider for a referral. Education can make a difference in your life and your health. ■

Other Professionals

Other specialists you may want to include on your personal diabetes team are:

- Dietitians who are trained in diet and nutrition and can help you develop meal plans and learn to count carbohydrates.
- Nurse Practitioners who provide direct care independently or in collaboration with a physician. They may be certified in specialties such as adult health, geriatrics, and diabetes. The initials BC-ADM indicate that the nurse is Board Certified in Advanced Diabetes Management.
- Pharmacists or druggists who dispense medications and may be specially trained in diabetes care.
- Foot doctors or podiatrists who provide routine foot care and treat foot sores, neuropathies and other foot problems resulting from your diabetes.
- Eye care specialists (ophthalmologists or optometrists), who treat retinopathy and other eye disorders that can result from diabetes.

- Psychologists, social workers, and psychiatrists who treat any emotional or psychological problems that you may have.
- Dentists who care for your teeth and gums, which are at high risk for disease because of your diabetes.

Over the course of your life with diabetes, you might also be referred to a cardiologist, nephrologist, neurologist, urologist or gynecologist. If you believe you would benefit from having any of these professionals on your team, ask your primary care provider for a referral.

Costs

Cost may be a concern when it comes to selecting health care providers. As with drugs and supplies, the rules will vary from one insurance company to another. Contact your insurance company before seeing any provider to be sure that the services are a covered benefit and to find out what you need to do to ensure reimbursement. Keep in mind that you *always* need to ask whether the health care provider will accept the amount that the insurer is willing to pay for a particular service, and, if not, ask in advance what the overage or any co-pay will cost. If your plan requires a referral from your primary care provider, be sure to arrange for this before seeing the specialist or entering the hospital.

All but a few states now require that health insurance companies cover diabetes education. However, many insurance companies and Medicare and Medicaid limit the number of hours of diabetes education or the specific programs they will cover. Many insurance companies will only cover programs that have been recognized by the American Diabetes Association. If your insurance will not cover the program, call the program and ask if there are scholarships available or what the cost will be for you.

Other commonly covered benefits are Medical Nutrition Therapy, as provided by a registered dietitian, and podiatry services, including any "special" shoes or orthotics designed for people with diabetic foot problems.

SELECTING A HEALTH CARE PROVIDER

If you need to choose a new physician or other health care professional, think back to what you particularly liked or disliked about those you've seen in the past. Ask trusted friends or health professionals for recommendations. Interview your professionals before signing on with them, since you may have different priorities than the person who referred you. Here are some of questions to consider when choosing a health care provider:

- Which providers does your insurance cover?
- Does the provider regularly stick to a schedule and see patients on time?
- How long do you have to wait from the time you call until an appointment is available?
- Does the provider regularly address psychosocial concerns and get to know patients as persons?
- Is the provider well-known in his or her field?

- Is the provider board certified?
- Does the provider stay up to date with the latest developments?
- What other professionals are available on the provider's staff?
- Are telephone calls returned promptly and is there someone available to call in an emergency?
- How many patients with diabetes does the provider normally treat?
- In which hospital does the provider have privileges?

Most of us feel somewhat intimidated when we go to a physician. We often feel judged or uncomfortable in raising concerns or questions. Take the time to select health care providers with whom you can enjoy a long term relationship. We find it amazing that most people spend more time and effort selecting a new car or television set than they do selecting a doctor or other health care professional!

Here are signs that you've found the right one:

- You trust the individual's expertise and recommendations.
- He or she shows a sincere and genuine concern for you as well as your diabetes, and expresses interest when you share information about your life, such as your family status and job situation. You feel that this provider can appreciate the additional challenges you may be facing.
- He or she makes you feel comfortable. You aren't afraid to raise any concerns, question a treatment recommendation, or ask for a referral.
- The provider realizes that communication is a two-way street, which involves listening as well as talking.
- The provider demonstrates that he or she is open to developing a true collaborative relationship with you.

With all health care providers, communication is the key to success. Remember that communication is a two-way street and involves both speaking and listening. Many people worry that their provider will be

How to Make the Most of an Office Visit:

It is true that physicians and other health care professionals have tighter schedules these days, so you may have a shorter office visit than you would like. That's why it's important to use the time wisely.

Make a list of your questions and decide what you want to accomplish before each visit. Some people find it helpful to keep a notebook at hand so that they can write down their questions as they think of them.

At the start of the visit, let your provider know that you have questions and concerns you need to address. Include concerns about your emotional state as well as your physical well-being. This is also the time to let your provider know about any new or worsening symptoms. Unless you tell your provider exactly how you feel, it will be very difficult for your provider to advise you about the appropriate treatment and refer you to others who can work with you.

While you need to be respectful of your provider's time, never ever be afraid to ask questions. There are no stupid ones. If your provider does not have the time or the answer, he or she can point you in the right direction. If you do not understand, keep asking until you do. It will be impossible for you to make wise decisions unless you understand fully what your choices are and what they can mean to you. Always feel free to raise your concerns, no matter how trivial they may seem. At the end of the visit, ask if you can repeat back what you understood. At the same time, let your provider know your goals, what you are willing and are not willing and able to do. And don't forget to remove your shoes and socks.

Some common questions are:

- *How do you think I am doing?*
- *Are there other approaches I should consider?*
- *Should I see a specialist?*
- *Are there additional tests I should have?*

- *What can I do to feel better?*
- *How can I use my monitoring results?*
- *What kind of records should I keep and how do I use them?*
- *What can I do to deal with my negative feelings about diabetes?*
- *I am really struggling with all there is to do. Can you help?*

insulted if they offer information that is not requested or ask for referrals to other health professionals. Some people believe that their physician should know how they feel and which questions to ask. But, as you have read, diabetes is managed primarily by you. Rather than accepting that your place is to follow orders, it is crucial to develop a relationship with your provider that is a true collaboration and partnership.

If you have tried but have not been able to create an effective partnership with your health care provider, consider finding another one with whom you can better relate.

COORDINATING YOUR CARE

As quarterback, one of your tasks is to be sure that all of your professionals are well informed about what the others are recommending. In an ideal world, your providers would consult with each other, but you cannot always count on that occurring. Be sure to let all of your providers know the medications you are taking and any changes in your health or therapies for other health problems, whether they are acute or chronic. Also be sure to have all of your prescriptions filled at the same pharmacy, which makes it more likely that the pharmacist will discover any potential adverse drug interactions before filling your new prescription.

Keep in mind that it is your health at stake. Your team members cannot make you adhere to a plan you do not want or are not able to follow. Remember that *you* make the choices.

— Mike Speaks —

The central role of the person who has diabetes was best illustrated at a recent community diabetes forum. I heard a woman who had type 2 diabetes for 6 years proclaim, "You can teach me, but you can't make me!" She went on to explain that only she had the power to manage her diabetes and that it was her responsibility to make sure that her healthcare professionals were all talking to one another about her care. After the program, I asked how she had come to that conclusion. She explained that after she was first diagnosed she had been taking multiple medications that were causing her to feel very depressed. Once she brought this to the attention of her various providers and insisted they consult with one another, her medications were adjusted and her depression went away. This experience taught her that she had to be the one to take charge. ■

FAMILY AND FRIENDS

Your friends and family members can be avid cheerleaders for you. They're likely to play an important role in your efforts to manage your diabetes. Just as with your health care providers, however, it is important that you and they realize that it is your diabetes, and not theirs.

— Gerri (Mike's wife) Speaks —

When Mike was diagnosed with diabetes, I knew nothing about the disease. I will never forget watching him give himself that first shot of insulin. I think it hurt me more than him. However, what hurt the most was learning that, for the first time, I could not make his illness better. When I asked his endocrinologist if I should learn how to give shots, he asked me whether I was going to be with Mike 24 hours a day, and told me he had to do this on his own. After fifteen years of sharing everything, this was not easy. I tried to be supportive by learning how to cook healthier foods and serving smaller portions, by reminding Mike that he should not be eating junk food when I caught him sneaking it, and by constantly asking what his blood sugar was. These attempts to share his illness only made Mike feel angry. It took some time before I realized that diabetes had not just changed our lifestyle, it had changed me. I had become a nagging spouse.

Eventually I realized that I was making things worse, and, while my intentions were honorable, they were not helping. I still cook healthier meals, but I no longer watch what Mike eats, nor do I ask what his meter is reading every time he checks. After all, it is his diabetes. I can only be there to provide support when he needs it. ■

Your diabetes affects your family and friends in many different ways. Aside from the daily demands, they will definitely be affected by your mood changes and other emotions. Diabetes may also be a source of worry for them because of their love for you. They may also be frightened about what the future holds.

Always remember, however, that your family and friends are not responsible for your having diabetes or for its management. Although you sometimes may be tempted to blame them for your disappointing results, your decisions are your responsibility and not theirs.

Many people with diabetes get great strength and support from their friends and family. Others, however, feel that their families add to their feelings of anger and frustration or even sabotage their efforts.

In order for your family and friends to provide meaningful support for you, it is essential that they learn about diabetes and, in particular, about your diabetes. This book may be an excellent starting point for them as well. If you are seeing a diabetes educator, ask whether your family can join you, if you feel that would be helpful. They also might want to attend classes and other programs at your local hospital that may include topics designed especially for family members.

When conflict arises about your diabetes, it is often because of a difference in expectations. Once more, clear and open communication is key. Share your diabetes game plan with your family and friends so that they know what you are trying to do and why. Ask them about their expectations of you. When your expectations mesh, it is easier for them to support your efforts. If you choose not to share this information, they can only guess. Most often, they will be wrong.

Don't hesitate to let your friends and family members know when they say or do things that bother you. At the same time, invite them to tell you when you say or do things that trouble them. Some friends and family members see themselves as enforcers of your diabetes plan—the so-called "diabetes police." If this is the kind of help you need, then, by all means, tell them. However, if it bothers you, be sure to let them know. In either case, keep in mind that they are probably trying to help the best way they know how.

If religion is a source of strength for you, you also may want to include your minister,

— Marti Speaks —

Some people with diabetes complain that well-intentioned family members and friends take it upon themselves to enforce what they believe to be the "proper diet." A story I heard from a colleague illustrates this point. As one of his patients reached for a brownie, her husband said, "Now dear, are you sure you want to eat that?" She responded, "Yes"- and took two brownies. ■

priest, or rabbi on your diabetes care team. Some people say they find clergy to be particularly helpful counselors for coping with the many different emotional issues they are facing. Another source of support can be from other people with diabetes. Many find it beneficial to share their diabetes struggles and triumphs with someone who has had similar experiences.

Keep in mind that diabetes does not just affect you physically, but also emotionally. And your emotions not only affect you, but also those around you. Of course, you are entitled to feel however you do. You do not have to downplay or change your feelings for other people. Just be aware of their effects on your family and friends. Put yourself in their place and try to understand their reactions to your feelings, just as you want them to understand and accept yours.

COMMUNITY

Another important component of the team is each of the different communities in which you live and work. As we mentioned earlier, the federal and many state governments have enacted legislation that requires minimum health insurance protections for people with diabetes. Other major federal laws that have proved helpful for patients are the Americans with Disabilities Act and the Equal Employment Opportunity Act, and many states have parallel statutes patterned after these laws. In addition, there are legislative initiatives designed to protect school children who have diabetes. Many of these laws came about as a result of the advocacy efforts of volunteers working with the ADA

(American Diabetes Association) and other concerned groups, but there is still a lot of work to do and sometimes enforcement becomes a problem. Through its advocacy programs, the ADA regularly arranges for legal representation of persons who have been discriminated against in the workplace or the public school systems. If this has happened to you, be sure to contact your local ADA office or the national office at 1-800-DIABETES.

Also, more and more employers are beginning to sponsor wellness programs for their employees that will help them to focus on lifestyle changes they wish to make. If no such program is available in your job, you may want to consider proposing it as a means for your employer to contain health insurance costs. You also should be sure to point out when your company-sponsored insurance does not provide coverage you need for your diabetes. Often, they may not even be aware of the problem and can find more acceptable alternative policies at no additional cost.

A Special Message for Family and Friends

Your support and encouragement are often critical for your loved one's success. You can be most supportive if you learn as much as you can about diabetes and communicate openly and freely with him or her. You also need to share your worries and concerns. Diabetes affects your life and future as well. Remember, however, that it is not your diabetes. You cannot manage or control it. You cannot change your loved one or his or her response to diabetes. Above all, be patient with each other as you work to define your roles and how together you will each live with and incorporate diabetes into your lives and relationship. ■

CHAPTER 5:
Know Yourself

How many times have you heard a quarterback or other professional athlete attribute success to playing within his "self?" Have you ever thought about what that really means? In simple terms, playing within your self means playing within your own capabilities, both physical and emotional. It requires that you believe in your ability to accomplish stated goals, with the help of your teammates and the other resources available to you.

Just as the quarterback about to throw a pass has to believe that he can get the ball to the receiver, he also has to believe that the receiver will be there to catch it. The successful quarterback makes it his business to know his own capabilities, as well as the strengths and weaknesses of his teammates and opponents. In earlier chapters, we provided information to help you know your "opponent" diabetes, as well as your "teammates" of family, friends, and health care team professionals. This chapter is devoted to getting to know yourself.

Before you can take charge of your diabetes, you need to make an honest assessment of your own strengths and any practical limitations that could affect how you take care of your diabetes. That's the only way to devise an effective game plan and play within yourself. Don't set yourself up for failure by assuming you will be able to do everything that is suggested. Remember that you are the same person, with the same pressures that you had before your diagnosis.

There are a number of factors that can influence your ability to care for your diabetes, such as your genes, your personality, or even the amount of travel your job requires. As you read about each factor described below, think of how it applies to you. The point is not to change anything in these areas; in some cases you can't. The goal is simply to help you understand how each of these affects you and the relative strength of these factors so you can develop a workable LIFE plan.

Although we discuss each factor individually, none of them exist in isolation. It is the combination of these factors that defines you and the way you approach your diabetes.

GENES

One of these factors is your genetic make-up. It is easy to blame your diabetes and your ability to care for it on your genes, as if there is nothing you can do about it. But that thought can be self-defeating. Your physical make-up does not determine whether you can care for your diabetes. It just affects what you may need to do. For example, there is a genetic component to weight. Just like type 2 diabetes, being overweight tends to run in families. We all know people who can eat anything and not gain an ounce. Others find it much more difficult to lose pounds and maintain their preferred weight. If you fall into this group, it does not mean that you cannot lose weight; it only means that it may be more challenging for you. The plan you create needs to take that into consideration, for example, by including diet and exercise in your plan to lose and maintain your weight. You may have to eat less and exercise more than someone without this predisposition.

The following questions can help you identify any genetic factors you need to consider in creating a plan to manage your diabetes:

- Does diabetes run in your family?
- Do members of your family tend to have a particular body type?
- Do members of your family tend to be overweight?
- Are there any other physical or emotional problems that are common in your family?

REAL-WORLD ISSUES

Real-world issues include your job, your family, and other priorities in your life. For example, if you travel as part of your job, you need to figure out how to handle staying in hotels, eating in restaurants, and other "on the road" situations that could affect your plan. There also may be periods when the needs of your family take priority over your own, such as when a family member is ill, is experiencing a job loss or a divorce, or is going through some other personally difficult time. These are often temporary situations, but at the time they occur, they are very real to you.

Finances are another significant factor. Diabetes can be very expensive. Not everyone can afford the medicine or the monitoring supplies. Perhaps your budget makes membership in a gym, or the purchase of certain foods, out of the question. Be sure to consider your finances when devising your plan. As we discussed earlier, health insurance coverage (including Medicare and Medicaid) varies among insurers. Make sure you know what your insurance covers and what it does not, and tell your health care providers about any limitations in your coverage or other financial concerns. They may be able to help you find another way to get what you need so you won't incur any additional costs.

— Marti Speaks —

I often meet patients who cannot afford their medicines or the monitoring supplies they need. Sometimes they choose not to fill a prescription but do not tell their provider. This is another situation where honesty is the best policy. Often, providers are able to prescribe a less costly medicine. If you can only afford a certain number of medicines, ask your provider whether there are some medicines that can be eliminated or replaced with cheaper alternatives. Many pharmaceutical companies have programs to provide medications at low or no cost for people who cannot afford them. There is information about these programs on the company websites; however, most require a referral from your provider in order to take advantage of them. ■

The following questions can help you identify some of the other real-world issues that may influence how you care for your diabetes:

• Does your job interfere with your ability to

manage your diabetes? For example, do you have time to monitor your blood sugar? Do you need to travel frequently?

- Do you often attend attend social events?
- What are your family responsibilities? Do family obligations or expectations interfere with your ability to manage your diabetes? Is your family interested in learning about diabetes and supporting your efforts to manage it?
- Do you have a safe place to walk or do other physical activity?
- Do you eat away from home or travel frequently?
- Do you have difficulty paying for your diabetes medicines or supplies? Do you have access to, and the financial means to buy, fresh fruits and vegetables and other foods?

PERSONALITY

Scientists are uncertain how much of your personality is based on genetics and how much on life experiences. Regardless, these factors have a great deal of influence on who you are and how you define yourself. Because personalities are established early in life, they are very hard to change. The point is to be aware of how your personality influences your approach to diabetes.

For example, you may consider stubbornness to be part of your personality. Using this trait to stick with a plan can be a strength when you are trying to accomplish your goals. Being stubborn can also be a hindrance, however, if it makes it difficult for you to listen to advice from others. Similarly, if it is in your nature to take charge of situations, that trait can be an asset or a detriment in managing your diabetes, depending on how you use it.

When thinking about your strengths and weaknesses, keep in mind the role that willpower plays in diabetes self-management. Many people think that if they just had "willpower" they could accomplish anything they wanted. They look at others who have made changes in their lives and think, "If only I had as much willpower as they do." However, there is no willpower gene. Willpower comes from knowing your self and staying committed to the path you have chosen.

The following questions can help you identify the effects of your personality traits on how you will manage your diabetes.

- How would you describe your personality?
- What are your dominant personality traits?
- How will these traits influence how you care for your diabetes?
- Can any of these traits be applied in a more positive way to help you manage your diabetes?

CULTURE AND RELIGION

Some of our cultural and religious beliefs have a very specific influence on diabetes care, such as the foods we eat or the holidays we celebrate. Others are more elusive, such as beliefs about health and illness, the roles our families play in our lives, and how we view our roles within our families. These beliefs can also influence the way we express our emotions. Part of knowing yourself is recognizing these influences and how they affect you. For example, religious beliefs and family support can be a great source of comfort and help. If you believe that the needs of your family come before your own, or that talking about feelings is a sign of weakness, it may be more difficult for you to ask for help in caring for your diabetes. You may tend to neglect your needs to care for others.

The following questions can help you identify how your culture and religious practices influence how you will care for your diabetes:

- Which of your cultural beliefs and practices influence how you manage your diabetes?
- Do any of your religious beliefs and practices influence how you manage your diabetes?
- Are there certain foods or activities that are part of your cultural or family traditions and celebrations that you need to incorporate into your planning?
- Are there essential foods or activities, such as fasting, that are a part of your religious rituals or celebrations that you need to incorporate into your planning?

EMOTIONS

Part of knowing yourself is being aware of your emotional response to diabetes. As the DAWN Study confirmed, the feelings you have can strongly influence your ability to care for your diabetes. As with all of the other factors, understanding your feelings can help you use them for your benefit, rather than allowing them to negatively affect you. The first step is to recognize them.

Common responses people have to their diabetes are denial, anger, guilt, fear, frustration, and sadness. Some experts believe that people work through these stages and finally come to accept the reality of their diabetes. While this is true to some extent, it is rarely that simple or straightforward. Most people experience all of these feelings at times and to different degrees over time.

Denial

Denial is a common reaction to bad news, like a diagnosis of diabetes or one of its complications. It is helpful at first because it allows you to filter the bad news until you are more able to handle it. However, if denial continues for a long period of time, it can be harmful. If you believe that you do not really have diabetes, that it is not really serious or that the complications will or will not happen no matter what actions you take, you may make decisions that are not in your best interest over the long term.

Anger and Guilt

Many people are angry that they developed diabetes or its complications. They may blame their parents for bad genes or wonder "why me?" Or they may feel angry with themselves for not having taken better care of their health, which in turn can lead to feelings of guilt and remorse. When people develop a complication, they may spend a lot of energy thinking "If only I had..." Over time, anger can cause feelings of sadness, helplessness, hopelessness, and even depression. It is difficult to believe in yourself or even have the confidence to manage your diabetes when you feel powerless.

Fear

Another emotion that can have a dramatic impact is the fear of not being able to do things you were able to do before. For example, you may worry you will not be able to provide or care for your family. You may also be afraid of developing complications from your diabetes or of experiencing low blood sugar reactions. As with the other emotions, fear is neither bad nor good. Fear can be a powerful motivator or can stand in the way of your ability to think and act clearly.

Frustration

As you deal with and manage your diabetes, it is common to be frustrated. Despite your best intentions and efforts, your blood sugar levels will at times be unpredictable. What worked yesterday may not work today, because there are factors other than your efforts that can influence your blood sugar levels. The key thing is not to let your frustration cause you to stop trying. Remember that it is not what you do at a particular moment that counts as much as what you do *most of the time*. Not every play can be expected to result in a touchdown!

Acceptance

Not all emotions related to diabetes are negative. For example, as you learn to manage your diabetes, you will feel a sense of accomplishment when you acquire new skills or get closer to your goals. Congratulate yourself when this happens — not for the result, but for all of the hard work it took to get there.

It is easy to misunderstand the concept of acceptance. Accepting the reality of diabetes does not mean you like it or that you never feel frustrated or never wish it would go away. Instead, it means that you understand and acknowledge the feelings you have about your disease. It means that you have made peace with it. You feel comfortable with the decisions you make and are able to do the things you choose to do. It is the essence of empowerment and playing within your self.

This does not mean that you should always be upbeat, but it does require that you make a conscious effort to reflect on your feelings: how are they affecting you and how might you use those feelings to make things better? For example, can you channel your anger about having diabetes into energy for managing it better, or for becoming involved in diabetes causes?

It's important to pay attention to your emotional response to diabetes, and to talk to someone who is a good listener. Talking about your feelings can be one of the most therapeutic things you can do. As you listen to yourself talk, you often gain valuable insights about the cause of your feelings and how you can deal with them.

— Mike Speaks —

I remember the first time I heard an adult admit publicly that he hated having diabetes and was frustrated about having to manage it himself. He was the National Chair of the ADA at that time and someone I respected. When I heard him, a light bulb went off in my head. I had the very same feelings, but never realized they were shared by others. From that moment, it was much easier for me to openly express my own feelings about diabetes. ■

Emotions that get in the way of caring for your diabetes or doing the things you usually enjoy should not be ignored. People with diabetes often suffer from clinical depression or anxiety, which can interfere with their ability to make wise choices or carry them out. If you believe you may have depression or anxiety, ask your health care team for help. Your primary care provider is a good place to begin. We know from research that counseling or medications do work, and what works best for most people is a combination of counseling and medication. Understanding your emotions will help you better manage your diabetes. The following questions can be useful for identifying how your emotions influence your actions:

- How did you feel about your diabetes when you were first diagnosed? How do you feel about your diabetes now?
- Which emotions would you use to describe your response to diabetes?
- Are any of your emotions interfering with managing your diabetes?
- What strategies have you tried for over-

coming your negative feelings?
- Can any of your emotions be used in a more positive way?
- What will it take for you to use your emotions more effectively?

PERSONAL PREFERENCES

There are some things you like to do better than others, and some things you just hate to do. Likes and dislikes are usually based on past experiences. If you are like most people, you will tend to gravitate toward activities you succeeded at in the past, while shying away from those where you were less than successful. For example, you may have had past experiences with exercise and dieting that color your feelings about your ability to start a new exercise program or diet. Your feelings are real and should be taken into account.

On the other hand, be careful not to underestimate your abilities. Just because you could not do something before, or did not like it, does not mean that you will have the same experience this time. It is okay to try something new and test the limits of your abilities.

The following questions can help you identify how your personal likes and dislikes influence how you will care for your diabetes:

- Do you enjoy doing any of the things you are considering in creating your self-management plan?
- Do you dislike doing any of the things you are considering in creating your self-management plan?
- Is there anything you can do to overcome this dislike?
- Are there other ways you can accomplish the same goal that are more consistent with your preferences?

PHYSICAL

Knowing your physical strengths and limitations is just as important as knowing your preferences, or making the effort to be emotionally self-aware. If you have a history of heart disease, for example, you do not want to begin an exercise program before consulting with your provider about what you can do safely.

As you live with diabetes, you undoubtedly will become more attuned to your own body and learn the warning signals that tell you things are out of balance. In most cases, you will be able to sense when your blood sugar levels are high or low by recognizing the symptoms discussed in Chapter 3. When you feel that your levels are changing, use your meter to take a reading. The meter can be very valuable in confirming that your feelings are correct.

— Mike Speaks —

The longer I live with my diabetes, the more conscious I am of how my body is responding, and I can sense my highs and lows. I always check my suspicions with my glucose meter, however, as it's still easy to be fooled. Sometimes I feel tired just because I am tired, and not because my blood sugar is high!

You can also use your blood glucose meter to learn about your physical responses to food, exercise, and stressful events. When you check your blood sugar, take the time to think about what the reading means and what could have caused the result. Ask yourself if the reading is what you expected or what might have caused it to be different. Understanding more about your body and how it responds will help you to use your power. Be honest with yourself and use what you learn to understand your physical responses, not to criticize your efforts. Share this information with your health care providers so they can better help you come up with an effective LIFE plan.

The following questions can help you identify how your health concerns or conditions influence how you will care for your diabetes:

- How do you feel when your blood sugar levels are high? Low? On target?
- Do you have other health conditions you are managing along with diabetes?
- How will these affect your ability to do what you want to do?
- How will your treatment plan affect other physical conditions you have?

KNOWLEDGE IS POWER

Remember, again, that all of the learning you do about diabetes can only teach you about diabetes as a disease or about other people's experiences with diabetes. It will not necessarily be what is real *for you*. Therefore, it is critical that you not only learn about dia-

— Mike Speaks —

I have probably learned the most from associating with other people who have diabetes or know more about the disease than I do. For me, that came through my involvement with the American Diabetes Association. At meetings and other events, it was very common for others to check their blood sugar and give themselves a shot at the same time, which made me much more comfortable doing it myself. Diabetes was discussed openly without embarrassment. The people with diabetes and the health care professionals that I have met continue to be a great help and support for me. ■

betes, but that you think about how this information fits with your life. You can then use what you learn to make choices that will be real and meaningful for you. It is through knowing yourself that you can create a self-management plan that fits your capabilities and discover the extent of your power to manage your diabetes

A Special Message for Family and Friends

Diabetes clearly has an emotional effect on the person who has it, which you will undoubtedly see in your loved one's moods and attitudes, and can even affect the way he or she acts toward you. Diabetes takes a similar emotional toll on family members and friends. Not only will your own worries and concerns affect you, but you may also be affected by your reactions to your loved one's moods and attitudes. Open and honest communication can go a long way to ease some of the tension. The same sources of support that are available to your family member could also be beneficial for you. ■

Part II: Doing

CHAPTER 6:

Making Decisions

Since you are still reading, we assume you want to be as healthy as possible and take charge of your diabetes. In Part I, you learned more about diabetes and yourself. Part II will help you adopt an overall strategy and give you the knowledge and skills you need to be successful with the other three LIFE steps for living with diabetes. Part III is about helping you manage your diabetes into the future.

As we have said previously, every day you face many choices about what you will eat, whether you will exercise, and how often you will check your blood sugar level. Having read Part I of this book, you may feel ready to make those choices. It has been our experience that you will find these choices much easier to make if you have an overall strategy in mind.

This overarching strategy is based on three

guiding principles: Role, Flexibility, and Targets. Identifying these principles will become the foundation upon which you will build the rest of your plan. Remember that the daily choices you make are the means to achieve your goal, not the goal itself. One of the reasons people struggle with making daily choices is because they are not quite sure what they are trying to accomplish. When you lose sight of your overall goal, it is much harder to keep working and stay motivated. That's where the guiding principles come in.

YOUR ROLE

In health care, the role of decision-maker has traditionally belonged to the physician or other health care professional, and not the patient. This works fine for acute illnesses. When you have an earache, for instance, you expect your physician to diagnose it correctly and prescribe the right medicine. Your goal is straightforward; you want the infection to clear up, and the pain to go away. Your role is to follow the recommended course of treatment.

But with diabetes, it's not that simple. The goals are not always that clear. Even worse, the recommended course of action may require you to make lifestyle changes you don't want—or find too difficult—to make. And this can put you at odds with your health

— Marti Speaks —

We all want other people to think well of us. Many people with diabetes tell me how much they dislike being weighed at their clinic visits and judged by what the scale says. Other people admit to adjusting the numbers in their blood sugar records to avoid criticism. While this is understandable and probably due in large part to how many health professionals respond, this is NOT a solution because it hides the problem rather than solving it. It's more effective to let your providers know what you think of the readings. Tell them you are doing the best you can and ask for help to solve the problem. ■

care professionals who expect you to be "compliant" or "obedient" with their instructions. If you think your job as a patient is to follow orders, you may feel embarrassed or frustrated if your efforts fall short of what was expected. You may feel uncomfortable about going to your next appointment because you feel like a naughty child.

Perhaps the best definition for "non-compliance" or "non-adherence" is two people working toward different goals. If you have ever had that experience at work or home, you know that it usually ends with everyone feeling tense and frustrated. That is the way much of health care used to be for people with diabetes. Both they and their professionals were working as hard as they could, but neither was reaching what they understood the goal to be.

Empowerment offers another way to approach these issues. One of the decisions you need to make is which aspects of your diabetes care you will control and which you will defer to your health care team. If you feel comfortable with your professionals making all the decisions, then tell them.

Your job, then, is to do exactly what they recommend for you. That works well for some people, especially when diabetes is new, but not as well for others. As long as you are making the conscious decision to defer to providers, you are not giving up your power. You are still the one in charge.

On the other hand, some people with diabetes choose to call some or all of the shots. If you decide that you want to be the primary decision-maker, by all means, tell your health care professionals. They can be most effective when they know how you want to be treated, what you want to accomplish, and how hard you are willing and able to work to reach your goals. It will be more productive for you and them.

One area that many people decide to defer to their health care provider is the choice of medications. Nevertheless, even if you accept the advice of your provider, you still have a responsibility to take the medication at the prescribed times and learn all that you can learn so that you can use it safely and most effectively. In addition, there are many different options for treating diabetes. If you feel that the medications you were prescribed are not working, talk to your health care provider, diabetes educator, or pharmacist about newer therapies or other options you could try. At the end of the day, it is your body and your life, and ultimately your responsibility.

It is possible that you will encounter some resistance from your health care providers when you begin to take charge of your diabetes. While many health care professionals have recognized and implemented a patient-centered approach to care, others have not. And even those who have may apply it in varying degrees. You may find that he or she is uncomfortable with a particular choice you have made, rather than your desire to take on the role of creating your treatment plan. If that's the case, you may be able to overcome your provider's resistance by learning as much as you can about your preferred option and asking questions so that you can make an informed decision. But if the provider expresses discomfort with your desire to be the decision-maker, you may need to find a new one.

— *Marti Speaks* —

When Bob Anderson and I first started talking with our colleagues about patient empowerment, we met a great deal of resistance. Some health professionals seemed to think that if they did not tell their patients what to do, their patients would simply be lost or even worse, go hog-wild in the cookie aisle in the grocery store. A common response was, "My patients expect me to tell them what to do." Our response was, "Did you ever ask them?" Other health professionals would say, "But you are asking us to give up control of our patients," to which we responded, "No, we are merely asking you to give up the belief that you are in charge." Fortunately, there is much less resistance today and more health professionals and people with diabetes are now embracing this approach. ■

FLEXIBILITY

As we said earlier in Chapter 2, you need to decide how much flexibility you want and need in your life. You can then tailor your plan to accommodate your decision. At one extreme, some people find it easier to follow a strict plan where they eat the same foods in the same amounts and exercise at the same time every day. Others want the absolute ability to change their mealtimes, menus, and exercise routine to suit their own schedule. Neither approach is right nor wrong, and there are many ways of handling diabetes in between these two extremes. The choice is up to you.

Deciding on the level of flexibility you need requires you to know yourself. You know whether you like having a detailed schedule or think of yourself as a free spirit. Perhaps you prefer a more structured program; you find that the fewer choices you have, the better you do. Alternatively, you may be more comfortable counting carbohydrates at every meal and balancing your food with medications and physical activity. No

— *Mike Speaks* —

Two shots a day never worked well for me. My work requires substantial travel (often through multiple time zones) and many late nights at the office. Then there are all those lunches and dinners out. To compound things, holiday and family gatherings mean many meals with high-carbohydrate ethnic foods that I really like. By taking a single shot of long-lasting insulin and bolusing with the fast-acting stuff before each meal, I gained the flexibility to accommodate my lifestyle much better and dramatically lowered my A1C levels. I now use an insulin pump and am able to achieve even better results. ◼

matter what approach you take, your level of responsibility is the same.

Two things to consider when you are making this decision are your schedule and your eating habits. If your daily life is pretty consistent and you are comfortable with that schedule, then you may not need a great deal of flexibility. If you never know from day to day or even hour to hour what you will be doing, you may decide that you want and need a lot of flexibility in your plan.

As with other things in diabetes, the amount of flexibility you want is not an all-or-nothing proposition. For example, some people have a pretty constant schedule during the week, but want more flexibility on the weekends so they can sleep later and eat at different times. They may have one plan for weekdays and another for weekends. Other people find that the timing and the food they eat for breakfast and lunch are pretty regular, but they want more flexibility at dinner. Others decide to make adjustments only for special occasions, such as holidays and vacations.

Although this is your decision, the members of your health care team can help. They often know "tricks of the trade" so that you can have the flexibility you need and still reach your goals. Keep in mind that more flexibility can often mean more work, more monitoring, more medications or shots, and more planning.

Once you have identified how much flexibility you want, and the role you will play, you have another major decision to make. The third major decision involves the blood sugar and other targets you want to reach. Although it is important to make these decisions from the very beginning, you can change your mind about one or all of them as you live with diabetes and gain more experience.

TARGETS

In Chapter 3, you read about the recommendations for blood sugar, blood pressure, and cholesterol. Meeting these targets can lower your risk for complications. These recommendations are based on solid research, and the textbooks make a strong case for striving to reach these levels. Many people with diabetes decide to play the odds and aim for the best blood sugar, blood pressure, and cholesterol levels possible. Others decide to start by first bringing their blood sugar levels closer to normal. They believe this is a more realistic goal. Still others decide they are doing all that they are willing or able or can afford to do and decide not to do anything differently. Identifying your targets will give you a better chance for achieving them. Regardless of your decision, be sure to tell your health care team what it is.

As you decide on your goals, think of these levels as targets rather than absolutes. Just as not every play results in a touchdown, you will not always hit your targets. There is no such thing as perfection in a football game or diabetes. Because there are so many factors that can affect your blood sugar, even when you do everything exactly the same, your blood sugar will not always be the same. If perfection is your goal, you most likely will fail and become frustrated. Aim for your target, but do not count on hitting it every time. As with many things in life, it is what you do most of the time that counts.

However, if you find that you are often not reaching your targets, do not wait until your next appointment with your provider to address this problem. Call and let him or her know that things are not working as hoped. Adjustments can often be made over the phone. If you wait two or three months until your next appointment, you are increasing your risk for complications.

Identifying your targets will lead to many other choices. There are a lot of options for reaching your blood sugar, blood pressure, and cholesterol goals, such as changing your eating or exercise habits, losing weight, deciding how often you will check your blood sugar, how you want to use monitoring information, or whether you will take pills or injections.

If your overall strategy is to keep your blood sugar as close to normal as you can, you will probably need to manage your diabetes more intensively. The more intensively you manage your diabetes, the more decisions you will have to make. The more choices you are willing and able to make, the more flexibility you will have.

As you can see, real diabetes is never as simple as in the textbooks. *Real diabetes is not easy.* You may have already decided where you stand when it comes to role, flexibility and targets. If you are struggling with any of those decisions, the following strategies can help you to either make these decisions or evaluate whether the guiding principles you chose will actually work in your life.

PRIORITIES

People today often feel that they are being pulled in different directions. We want to make our families, our jobs, our health, our faith, our friends, and time for ourselves top priorities. No matter how important these are, they cannot all be the top priority all of the time.

Your priorities are influenced by what you value. Health, security, love, faith, family, and career success are examples of values. The more you value something, the more motivated you are to achieve a good result in that area. If your number one value is your family, for instance, you are probably very motivated to spend time with your children and grandchildren. You make it a priority in your life and are willing to give up other things in order to have that time. Priorities reflect the level of importance you place on your values.

Caring for diabetes takes time. The more intensively you manage it, the more time and energy it takes. As you create your plan, think about your priorities. Rate them from 1 to 10, with 1 being the most important. Here are some questions that can help:

- As you look at your list, think about what is *truly* important to you.
- Are there conflicts?
- Do your priorities match these values?
- Where does caring for your diabetes fall on that list?
- What choices do you need to make about your diabetes to be consistent with your values?
- How does the priority you placed on caring for your diabetes fit with your other priorities?

There are no right or wrong answers to these questions. The point is to understand your priorities, not necessarily to change them.

Over the course of your life with diabetes, you may find that your priorities change. If you are struggling with a particular goal, do not be afraid to question whether it is truly a priority for you.

COSTS AND BENEFITS

One way to make decisions is by weighing the costs, or negatives, and benefits, or positives, of your alternatives. Whenever you make a choice, you usually have to give up something in order to gain something else. Most of us have looked at other people's lives and wondered why they do not take steps to change their situation. Often it is because they feel that the comfort of keeping things the same outweighs what they will sacrifice in making a change.

The decisions you make about caring for your diabetes also have costs and benefits. Choosing to bring your A1C level into your target range or losing weight means that you may have to give up things you enjoy to reach your goal. Often when you give things up, you defer immediate gratification to gain a long-term benefit. For example, you may need to give up some food you enjoy today in order to be healthier tomorrow. Or you may need to give up time doing other things in order to have time to exercise.

Another idea is to list the costs of a decision on one side of a piece of paper and the benefits on the other. As you review your list, the question to ask is "Is it worth it to me?" "Is what I will gain worth what I will give up?" If the answer is "yes," then you are ready to make a commitment. If the answer is "no," you may not be ready to make a decision. You might also ask what it would take to make it worthwhile for you. This can help you to understand what will tip the balance for you. It is a good idea to keep your list. When it feels like you are struggling or not getting anywhere, pull out your list as a reminder of the benefits you hoped to achieve.

FEELINGS

As we discussed in Chapter 5, choices are influenced by feelings. Your emotional response to diabetes influences your decisions and behavior, and can affect your ability to stick with your plan. When you feel angry, you are likely to make a different choice than when you are calm. Negative feelings are not a sign of weakness nor are they necessarily bad. Not wanting to feel guilty about your choices, or making choices that will help eliminate other negative feelings, can be an additional reason for making a change.

TALKING WITH YOUR HEALTH CARE TEAM

Once you have made decisions about your role, how much flexibility you want in your self-management plan, and what targets you want to reach, have a conversation with your health care team and explain what you have chosen to do. It is easier to work together if you are all working toward the same goal. They can be most helpful to you when your guiding principles are clear to you and to them.

Many people are hesitant to have this type of discussion with their doctor. They worry that the doctor does not have time or is not interested in their opinion on these issues. They may think that the doctor should know what to ask or what they are thinking. But health professionals are only as good as their patients help them to be. This is not the time to be timid.

Starting the discussion is often the hardest part, so these "conversation starters" may help. Once the conversation is underway, be honest and straightforward about what you need or want. For example:

- "I need more flexibility with the timing of my medicine and meals, especially on weekends. Can you help me or refer me to an educator or dietitian who can help?"
- "Here is an article I read about a new medication for type 2 diabetes. Have you had any experience with it? Do you think it would work for me?"
- "You mentioned some of the benefits of this type of therapy. Are there any negatives? What are some other options?"
- "I am really struggling to reach the recommended target levels and I think it is more realistic for me to work toward an interim level for now. Are there one or two things I could do, or we could do together, to help me reach my target?"

Identifying your guiding principles gives you the foundation for how you will manage your diabetes. The next chapters will help you think about your day-to-day options and the skills you will need to implement your overall plan.

A Special Note for Family and Friends

It is critical for people with diabetes to take charge of their diabetes by identifying what role they are willing and able to assume for the design and implementation of their plan and how much flexibility they need in their lives. Both of these decisions involve serious reflection and honest assessment of their needs and capabilities. It is important that they fully embrace these decisions for them to be effective. You can help by sharing your thoughts on these issues. It is also important that you share your worries and concerns—such as how your schedule will be affected by the level of flexibility they choose.

When it comes to setting targets, the input of health care professionals is invaluable, but the targets have to be realistic as well. Identifying all of these things is ultimately the responsibility of the person with diabetes. Whatever those decisions, your support will play a key role in their success. ∎

IDENTIFY YOUR GUIDING PRINCIPLES

The following is a summary to help you identify you guiding principles.

Role

1	2	3	4	5	6	7	8	9	10

On a scale of 1 to 10, how much **responsibility** do you want for your plan?

Are there aspects of your plan for which you want total responsibility?

Are there aspects of your plan for which you want shared responsibility?

Are there aspects of your plan for which you want your health care provider to take responsibility?

Flexibility

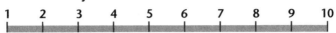

On a scale of 1 to 10, how much **flexibility** do you want in your plan?

Are there situations or times where you need more flexibility?

Are there situations or times where you want a more structured plan?

Targets

What are your **targets** for:

Blood sugar levels before meals

Blood sugar levels after meals

Blood sugar levels at other times

Blood pressure

Lipids: HDL; LDL; Triglycerides

Weight

Other

CHAPTER 7:

Making Choices

Now that you have decided on the role you want to take, the amount of flexibility you desire, and your targets, you have formulated your overall strategy. Congratulations. You are now ready to use these guiding principles to evaluate your options.

In this chapter, we will discuss how to create the specific elements of your diabetes plan. This is Step 3 of the four LIFE Steps—the "how" part of caring for your diabetes.

REACHING YOUR TARGETS

We have talked about the importance of setting targets for your blood sugar, blood pressure and cholesterol. Fortunately, many of the things you do to lower your blood sugar level will also help to lower your cholesterol and blood pressure.

The good news is that you have many options. The information starting on page 197 summarizes some of the different approaches. Knowing your options and thinking through the pluses and minuses will not only help you reach your targets but also help you to take charge of your diabetes care. In general, you have choices in each of the three major categories that make up the treatment options for diabetes. These are medications, lifestyle, and monitoring. They will constitute the basis of your plan for living with your diabetes.

Knowing and thinking about your options ahead of time will help you to be better prepared when you visit your health care team. It will help focus the visit around the specific issues that are important to you. Knowing your options also gives you greater power to make daily decisions that are consistent with your overall strategy and guiding principles.

If you have type 1 diabetes, insulin will be your primary treatment. There are, however, options about the types of insulin and number of injections. In addition, balancing lifestyle with insulin is a major part of your job.

If you have type 2 or pre-diabetes, you may choose to manage initially through meal planning and exercise. However, new guidelines call for the use of oral medications right from the start for type 2 diabetes and are sometimes used by people with pre-diabetes as well. Even if you are not interested in losing weight, you may still be able to lower your blood sugar levels through meal planning and exercise. Because a healthy diet and exercise benefit just about everyone, you might decide to choose these options even if they are not your primary treatment.

MEDICATIONS
Type 1 Diabetes

As we have said before, the treatment for type 1 diabetes is taking insulin along with meal planning and exercise. Once again, you have options from which to choose.

Although there is no substitute for insulin at this time, people with type 1 can choose to take two to four or more shots a day or to use an insulin pump. You may also be able to take inhaled insulin instead of giving yourself insulin shots or use one of the other injectable medicines along with insulin.

If your choice is to take two shots a day, you may not need to check your blood sugar as often, so this plan is easier and less costly. However, there are negatives to this approach as well. It may not be enough to reach the targets you have identified. Most people find that their blood sugar levels go up and down at different times throughout the day. They may have several highs and several lows and as a result feel tired and irritable much of the time. When your blood sugar changes often, your moods and emotions may change often as well. Most people say that they feel worse when their blood sugar is frequently going up and down than when it is more steady. People with type 1 who do reach their targets with two shots often find that they need to pay very strict attention to the time of their injections and when and what they eat. They still have to work hard to keep everything in balance.

People who take three or more injections per day are said to be managing their diabetes intensively. When people with type 1 diabetes take more shots and monitor more often, they are usually better able to reach and maintain their targets. They also have more flexibility in the timing and amount of food they eat and when they exercise. However, taking more shots definitely increases the cost and can be harder to do. Weight gain and low blood sugar reactions are more common among people who use intensive management. As your blood sugar comes down, you lose less sugar in your urine. The sugar in the urine contained calories that your body now has available. When you keep your blood sugar closer to the recommended level, you no longer have as far to drop to hit a low level. Relatively minor changes in your food or exercise can cause your blood sugar to fall too low.

Other options have to do with how you take your insulin. Many people find that using an insulin pen is more discreet and makes it

— *Gerri Speaks* —

Shortly after Mike's diagnosis, we were in a crowded restaurant. After a long wait, we placed our order and Mike took his insulin. However, a half hour later the food had not come, not even bread. Mike started to feel ill and stood up to go get some air. He stumbled as he got up from the table and passed out on the floor. I thought he was dead. It was the first time my husband had a severe low blood sugar reaction. Fortunately, there was a doctor in the restaurant who knew to ask if Mike had diabetes and what to do. Diabetes became very real to me that night. I learned not to panic, and Mike learned to wait to take his insulin until food arrives. ■

easier to take multiple shots a day. You do not have to draw up your dose, mix insulins yourself, or carry a vial and syringe. An insulin pump is a battery-operated device you wear that delivers a steady flow of insulin throughout the day and night. You push a button and take a bolus dose of insulin before each meal to match the amount of carbohydrates you are eating. Some people find that this gives them the best possible blood sugar levels and the greatest degree of flexibility. Others prefer to take shots because they do not like the idea of being attached to a device all the time. They often feel that it is a constant reminder of their diabetes or may interfere with intimate moments. Some people think a pump is more discreet while others believe that it draws more attention to their diabetes. Pumps are also costly to buy and operate. Before you consider a pen or a pump, be sure to check with your insurance company to find out if the costs are covered.

Type 2 Diabetes

The treatment for type 2 diabetes has traditionally been to start with lifestyle changes, usually meal planning and exercise, then to add one, two, or even three pills for diabetes and, ultimately, to add insulin or other injectable medications. But a growing recognition of the progressive nature of type 2 diabetes and the importance of keeping blood sugar levels close to normal has prompted some changes in that approach. Newer treatment guidelines for type 2 diabetes call for the use of an oral medication called metformin along with lifestyle changes from the time diabetes is diagnosed. Metformin is often used by people with pre-diabetes as well. When that is no longer enough to keep your blood sugar on target, the next step is to either add another type of pill, another injectable or insulin. It works better to add medicines because different types work differently. Combining two types of medicines is more effective than simply switching to a different type of pill. There is also a maximum dose at which oral medications are effective or safe. Adding to the dose past that point will not help you lower your blood sugar any further, which is another reason for adding additional types of medications that either work differently or will help your current medicine work better.

Needing more medicines does not mean that you failed; it simply means that you need more help to keep your blood sugar on target. Diabetes pills, insulin, and other injectables work well to lower your blood sugar. It is a matter of being patient and finding the right medicine or combination that works best for you.

Although you may start with lifestyle changes and oral medications, over time most people with type 2 diabetes will need insulin or other injections to keep their blood sugar levels within the target range. In fact, many people with type 2 diabetes are starting insulin earlier than in the past because of new evidence showing that starting sooner lowers the risk for complications. Most people find the idea of taking injections very upsetting. After all, no one gets excited about taking shots. It may help to know that insulin injections are not like the shots you remember from your childhood. The needles are small, thin, and almost painless. In fact, many people who start insulin claim with astonishment that taking an injection is less uncomfortable than doing a finger stick.

There are several other common concerns about insulin. Some people believe insulin causes complications, or even death. This is often based on what happened in the past to a family member or friend after they started taking insulin. It is more likely that person started insulin late in the course of his or her diabetes, either when he or she was very ill or already had developed complications. In reality, if insulin had been started sooner, these complications might have been avoided. Many people who eventually take insulin say they wish they had initiated it sooner because they feel so much better once they do.

— *Marti Speaks* —

I have taught many people to give themselves insulin shots over the years. I remember one woman in particular who had just retired from teaching and was looking forward to traveling with her husband. When she found out she had diabetes, she did everything she could to avoid insulin because she thought it would be a hindrance to their plans. She lost weight and began to exercise, but her blood sugar remained high. Just before they were to leave on a trip to Europe, she and her primary care provider decided she needed to start insulin. I taught her how to take shots the day before they left, and she was a quick learner. When she returned, she called to tell me she had a great trip and no problems with her insulin. She went on to tell me what so many other patients have said—that she did not know why she waited so long because she had so much more energy. A phrase I often hear is, "I did not know how bad I felt until I started feeling better." ■

Some people are worried about insulin reactions, especially if they live alone. They are afraid that taking insulin may cause them to lose some of their independence. This is a real issue, but many people find that with the newer insulins and frequent blood sugar monitoring, it is less of a problem than it used to be. Creating a safety system such as a panic button or a neighbor who calls to check every morning can also add to your peace of mind.

Another concern about taking insulin is gaining weight. Just like in type 1 diabetes, some people do gain weight when they begin taking insulin. Insulin works well to lower blood sugar levels and help your body use food more efficiently. In addition, as your blood sugar level comes down, you will lose less glucose in your urine. Your body now has those extra calories to use. So if you eat the same amount, you are likely to gain weight. If this is an issue for you, ask your provider for a referral to a certified diabetes educator or dietitian who can help you adjust your meal or exercise plans to prevent weight gain.

As you create your plan, there are several things to consider:

- What does it mean to me to take insulin?
- What am I most worried about?
- Am I afraid to take insulin? What about it scares me and why?
- How satisfied am I with my blood sugar levels?
- What benefits do I see in taking insulin?
- What questions do I need answered before I can decide if I will take insulin? For example, you may want to know about other options for treating diabetes.
- Do I know someone who recently started insulin I can talk with about his or her experience?
- What would have to change for me to consider insulin?

Making the move to insulin is a big step. If you have type 2 diabetes, most of the time you will have the chance to think about it and get your questions answered before you decide. As you make your decision, keep your targets and guiding principles in mind and ask yourself if insulin will help you attain your overall objectives.

Once you have decided to take insulin, then you have further choices about how many shots per day you will take, and what type or types of insulin, much like people with type 1 diabetes.

Multiple Medicines

Remembering to take your medicines can be difficult. The more times you take pills and the more pills you take, the harder it is to remember. Along with diabetes medicines, you also may be taking pills for your blood pressure, cholesterol, an aspirin and medicines for other health concerns. Be sure to let your providers know of everything you are taking—including vitamins, over-the-counter drugs or herbal supplements—so they can be aware of any possible adverse effects.

The average person with type 2 diabetes takes nine different medicines. It is costly and can be a real nuisance; but there are things you can do to make it easier:

- Choose a time to take your medicines, such as with a meal or at bedtime.

- Ask your doctor or pharmacist if there are any special precautions or side effects. If you have side effects, contact your health care provider rather than just stopping the medicine. It is not safe to stop some medicines abruptly.
- Ask your doctor or pharmacist why labels are included that say things such as "take with meals."
- Be sure to let your health care team know if you are having trouble paying for your medicines. They may not think to ask, but it is a common problem. They will not think less of you. In fact, they may be able to help with samples or introduce you to lower cost drug programs for which you qualify.
- Set up all your medicines in a container for the week. You can buy these for very little cost at almost every pharmacy. This also makes it easier to take them along when you go out to eat or travel.
- If you are not able or choose not to take a medicine or take it more or less often than prescribed, be sure to tell your providers. They need to know the facts to make informed decisions, too.

LIFESTYLE
Meal Planning

Because food affects your blood sugar, blood pressure, and cholesterol, meal planning is part of your plan regardless of which type of diabetes you have. Since the carbohydrates you eat raise your blood sugar level, many of the daily choices you make in caring for diabetes involve balancing the food you eat with your medicines and physical activity.

In spite of what you may have been told, there is no such thing as a "diabetic diet." No foods are strictly forbidden, and no foods are good or bad. Once again, it is about learning the options and making choices.

The four main reasons for meal planning are:

- Managing your blood sugar
- Managing your cholesterol and blood pressure
- Preventing and treating the complications of diabetes, including obesity, cardiovascular and kidney disease
- Keeping healthy and meeting your personal nutrition needs

One or more of these may be reasons for you to plan meals. Being clear about your reasons and how they fit into your overall strategy will make it easier to choose what and how much you will eat.

Once you know your reasons for meal planning, there are different approaches you can use. Some are simple (eating consistent meals at regular times) and others are more complex (counting carbohydrates). If you have never been to a dietitian, if it has been a long time since you met with your dietitian, or if your reasons for meal planning have changed, ask your provider for a referral. A dietitian can help you develop a meal plan that takes into account your usual eating habits, likes and dislikes, preferences and religious or cultural practices.

There are several key points that may make planning meals easier. The first is to realize that eating to manage your blood sugar level is different than following a weight-loss diet. Weight-loss diets are designed to be followed until you reach your weight goal. Once you go back to your usual eating habits, the weight often returns. But diabetes is a lifetime condition, and no one can follow a diet forever. You need to be able to use your meal plan in many different situations every day. The second thing to keep in mind is that the purpose of meal planning is to reach your targets, not to follow a diet.

You also need to consider that there are times you may decide to deviate from your plan. Some people call this "cheating." But what does that really mean? Whom are you cheating? In reality, you are merely making a choice to ignore your meal plan at that time, which is your right. Thinking of yourself as a cheater or feeling guilty can be self-defeating. If you are like most people, you will find it more useful to make a choice about how you will handle special events, holidays, or other situations ahead of time. Some options are:

- Choose to ignore your plan for that meal
- Eat small portions of foods you would usually avoid
- Take additional insulin

- Exercise more to balance your blood sugar
- If it is a "potluck," take food you enjoy that fits with your goals

There is no one right or wrong way to handle these situations. How you handle each one will probably be different. As you create your plan, however, you do need to consider these events. Be sure to take ownership of the decision and then to evaluate it based on the results. You are the only one who can decide if the choice you made was worth the results in terms of your overall strategy.

PREPARING FOR YOUR VISIT WITH THE DIETITIAN

There are some things you can do to prepare for your visit with the dietitian so that it is more productive. One is to write down everything you eat for one or two weekdays and a weekend day. This will help you use the time to your best advantage. In addition, food has meanings for most of us beyond nutrition. It often means love, comfort, family, culture, or traditions. Along with knowing your guiding principles and your reasons for meal planning, it also helps to know about yourself and your relationship with food. As you prepare for your visit or create your plan, think about your past experiences as you answer these questions about yourself:

- Have I ever tried to stay on a diet before? What helped my efforts? What got in the way?
- Have I ever lost weight only to regain it? Why did that happen?
- Are there foods that are so important to me that giving them up would be a real sacrifice?
- Are there foods I commonly eat when I am feeling blessed, stressed, or depressed?
- If I create a meal plan that does not include my favorite or comfort foods, will I feel deprived and give up?
- Are there foods that I can't stop eating once I start eating them?
- How will my family respond to my efforts? How would I like for them to respond?

Is there anything I can do or say that might cause them to respond in the way I prefer?
- When will using my meal plan be hardest for me? When will it be easiest?
- How will I handle sick days?
- How do I want to handle holidays or special occasions and events?

PHYSICAL ACTIVITY

Physical activity helps you look and feel better. Along with improving general health and fitness, physical activity has specific benefits for people with diabetes and pre-diabetes. Physical activity helps:

- Lower your blood sugar, your blood pressure, and your cholesterol levels
- Make cells more sensitive to insulin
- Coping with stress
- Burn calories
- Improve your appearance
- Improve fitness
- Increase your energy level

Studies have shown that the people who are able to maintain weight loss are those who exercise. If you have pre-diabetes, exercise along with weight loss helps to prevent or delay the onset of diabetes. Many people say they exercise because they feel so good when they stop. They feel relieved of some of their stress, more energetic, and more positive about themselves.

You have no doubt heard about these benefits before, but they may not have been enough to overcome your negative thoughts about exercise. Physical activity does not have to be about joining a gym or running for miles. In the DPP study, walking 30 minutes a day, 5 times per week helped to lower blood sugar levels and improve cardiac function. This is the same as the recommendation from the American Heart Association. This type of exercise does not have to be done all at once: 10 minutes three times a day is as effective as 30 minutes of activity. You may be able to reach this level of activity by changing some of your daily routines: parking further from the door, walking for short errands instead of driving, and taking a walk during coffee breaks and at lunch. The important thing is to do more than you do now.

You might find that wearing a pedometer to count your steps helps keep you motivated. It becomes a way to track your progress and challenge yourself to walk more. Building up to at least 10,000 steps or 5 miles, which takes most people about an hour, is the recommended target. If weight loss is part of your overall strategy, 60 minutes of walking or other exercise will probably be needed most days of the week. In order to sustain weight loss, you will probably need 60 to 90 minutes of daily activity.

Most adults have at one time started to exercise and then stopped. Exercise does take time and effort. One way to maintain your commitment to exercise is to choose something you like and will continue to do. If you enjoy dancing, put on your favorite music and move. Some people find that having someone to exercise with helps to increase their commitment and makes it more enjoyable. Another barrier to exercise that many people face is time. Our lives get busy, and we give up exercise to do other things. There is no one answer to these issues. Choosing something you like to do and knowing your priorities will help you make exercise part of your life.

— *Marti Speaks* —

Patients often ask me "What is the best exercise for people with diabetes?" I usually respond that the best exercise is the one you will do! ■

If you are considering exercise, the following questions may help you create a realistic plan:

- Have I ever started a physical activity program before? What helped my efforts? What hindered my efforts?
- What do I enjoy doing? What would make exercise more enjoyable for me?
- Is there a time of day when it will be easier to exercise? Am I a morning or night person?

- How can I adjust my routine to accommodate exercise?
- Are there specific activities I can do in good weather? In bad weather?
- Are there scheduling issues I need to discuss with my family?
- Would it help to exercise with a family member or friend?
- How involved would I like my family to be? Are there activities we could do together?
- How do I think my family will respond? How would I like them to respond? Is there anything I can do or say that might cause them to respond in the way I prefer?

Talk with your primary care provider, diabetes educator, or dietitian about your answers to these questions. They can offer ideas for how to exercise safely and how to get the most benefit from the time you spend.

TRACKING YOUR RESULTS

The quarterback knows right away if a play worked. You have the same ability in managing your diabetes. You can check your blood sugar at home using a drop of blood and a meter. These readings tell you how often your blood sugar is within your target range.

Checking your blood sugar is not something you do just to satisfy your health care team. It is hard to stay motivated to do something unpleasant when you feel you are doing it for someone else. Remember that you are checking for yourself—to get the information you need to make sound choices. Then consider how often you need to check so that you will have the information you need. Checking your blood sugar helps you take charge of your diabetes and make choices that are in keeping with your overall strategy.

It is easy to fall into the trap of thinking of your blood sugar number as a grade on a test or a judgment about whether you have been good or bad. Because you do not have control over everything that affects your blood sugar levels, it is more useful to think of these numbers as information. If your reading is not in the target range, ask yourself what is different. Be honest. Did you eat more or less than usual? Were you more or

— *Mike Speaks* —

There is no substitute for honesty in managing your diabetes. Clearly, you need to be accurate when reporting results and problems to your health care professionals. But honesty starts at home. It is tempting to blame others for poor results or ignore the facts when looking at blood sugar readings. When I am honest with myself, I can usually figure out why my results are what they are. ◼

less physically active than usual? Are you feeling ill or more stressed than usual?

There may be times when you will not be able to understand your readings. If this happens often, talk to your health care team about what could be causing the results. Be sure to take a record of your blood sugar levels and your meter to all of your provider and educator visits. Let them know what you think about the numbers, and ask what could have caused the highs and lows you cannot explain. If your number is often out of range, you probably need a change in your medica-

THE LITTLE DIABETES BOOK YOU NEED TO READ

tion or dose. Fortunately, there are more options for treating diabetes than ever before, so do not give up until you find the right one.

There are several things to consider as you think about checking your blood sugar level that can make it easier to develop a workable plan. These are:

- How many strips does my insurance company cover?
- How can I remember to check my blood sugar?
- How can I keep the supplies on hand and with me when I am away from home? Would it help to keep one meter at home and one at work?
- How will I handle checking my blood sugar when I am away from home? What situations will be common for me? (Consider, for example, how you will handle checking your blood sugar levels at work, or while in a restaurant with your family, a friend or a business associate.)
- How involved do I want my family to be? Do I want them to ask me about my numbers or wait until I tell them? How can I

— Mike Speaks —

When I first began checking my blood sugar level, my wife and children would always ask what my number was. Although I knew it was out of deep concern for me, it made me feel as if they were judging my performance. Once I explained my feelings, the questions stopped and I was much more comfortable letting them know when I needed their help. After all, it is still just a number to guide me in treating myself. ■

tell them what will be most helpful?

- How will I feel if I have a number out of my target range when I have been working as hard as I can to bring it down?
- What are some strategies I can use to keep myself feeling motivated when the numbers are not what I expected?

As you read earlier, the measure of long-term blood sugar levels is the A1C. When the members of your health care team talk about diabetes being out of control, they are usually referring to a high A1C level or blood sugar levels that go up and down often. They do not mean that you are out of control as a person. Although A1C readings are sometimes referred to as a report card, they are really just numbers that you and your health care team need to know so you can manage your diabetes effectively. Remember, your worth as a person is not reflected in your A1C level.

You can also use the questions listed above when you receive your blood pressure and cholesterol levels from your provider. Be sure to ask about your numbers and keep track so you get a better idea of how well your overall strategy is working. If your numbers are not in the target range you have set for yourself, ask your health care team what else can be done to improve them.

Keeping a record of your blood sugar levels can help you better understand your readings. Although most meters have a "memory" of recent results, there is no substitute for writing down your levels so that you can examine them more carefully. Although you may not want to write down your levels all of the time, there are times when it may be particularly helpful—for example when your numbers do not reflect your efforts, when your readings are often too high or too low and when you are ill or under more stress than usual.

As you look at your record, ask yourself:

- Is there a pattern or certain times or situations when my blood sugar levels are out of the target range more days than not?
- How do different foods affect my blood sugar levels?
- How does my activity affect my blood sugar levels?
- How does stress affect my blood sugar levels?
- What changes could I make in meal planning, exercise, medications or how I handle stress that might improve my blood sugar levels?

If your blood sugar level is frequently out of your target range and you need help to know how to make adjustments to change it, call your provider. Do not wait until your next appointment for a change in your therapy.

Use the list at the end of this chapter for ideas, or as a checklist of options you can use to make your LIFE plan for diabetes.

A Special Note for Family and Friends

There are a variety of options for managing diabetes. In spite of what you may have heard, there is no one right way or no one best way. There is no such thing as the best diet or foods you should or should not eat. One of the most important decisions your loved one needs to make is the strategies he or she will use to manage diabetes. Although there is always more that could be done, keep in mind that no one can do everything at once or all of the time. Perfection is neither possible nor expected. ■

OPTIONS FOR REACHING YOUR TARGETS

The following is a list of strategies you can use to improve your blood sugar, blood pressure and cholesterol levels, as well as to lose weight and quit smoking. You may find these ideas will help as you formulate your plan.

— *Blood sugar* —

TO LOWER MY BLOOD SUGAR I CAN:

Eat smaller portions

Eat smaller portions more often throughout the day

Eat fewer sweets

Maintain a reasonable weight

Be more physically active

Take medicine (diabetes pills, insulin or other medicines)

Take a different dose of medicine

Take a combination of medicines (diabetes pills, insulin or other medications)

Add or adjust insulin dose, timing or shots per day ■

— *Cholesterol* —

TO LOWER MY CHOLESTEROL I CAN:

Eat less saturated (hard) and trans fats and cholesterol-containing foods like butter, bacon, shortening

Maintain a reasonable weight

Eat skinless, lean meats

Be more physically active

Take medicine to lower cholesterol

Eat more soluble fiber, such as dark, green leafy vegetables and whole grain cereals

Use margarines and dressings with plant stanols/sterols added

TO LOWER MY LDL I CAN:

Eat less saturated (hard) and trans fats and cholesterol-containing foods like butter, bacon, shortening

Use monounsaturated oils instead of saturated fats

TO IMPROVE MY HDL I CAN:

Exercise more

Lower triglycerides

Use monounsaturated oils in place of saturated fats

Eat more baked or broiled cold-water fish

TO LOWER MY TRIGLYCERIDES I CAN:

Lower my blood sugar

Eat fewer sweets

Drink less sweet liquids (including unsweetened fruit juice)

Drink less alcohol

Eat more broiled or baked cold-water fish ■

— *Blood pressure* —

To LOWER MY BLOOD PRESSURE I CAN:

Eat less salt

Stop smoking

Take my blood pressure medicine

Change dose, number, or type of blood pressure medicine

Be more physically active

Maintain a reasonable weight ■

— *Weight* —

To LOSE OR MAINTAIN MY WEIGHT I CAN:

Eat smaller portions

Eat smaller portions more often throughout the day

East fewer sweets

Eat less fat

Eat a more balanced diet

Be more physically active ■

— *Smoking* —

<u>*To cut back and quit smoking I can:*</u>

Attend stop-smoking classes

Use nicotine patches, lozenges or gum

Take anti-smoking medicine

Smoke less often ■

Adapted with permission. © The University of Michigan, 2004

CHAPTER 8:
Making Changes

You have now shaped the overall strategy for managing your diabetes and considered some of the daily choices you need to make. You have identified your three guiding principles (Step 2) and formulated your plan (Step 3). Now comes the most challenging part—experimenting with and evaluating your plan (Step 4).

As you made your decisions in Steps 2 and 3, you probably selected some changes you want to make to achieve your targets; this is how you turn your plan into action. But just as football is a game of inches, so is making changes. One reason people struggle with making changes is that they try to do too much at one time and then get discouraged when their efforts fall short. When this happens, it is easy to lose confidence in your abilities and simply give up.

As every quarterback knows, not every play results in a touchdown. More often, success comes through the team plugging away down the field a few yards at a time until someone ultimately crosses the goal line. There are often setbacks; sometimes the team loses ground. You will undoubtedly have setbacks too. Like the quarterback, learn from your attempts and keep going.

As you begin this chapter, it may be helpful to think about a past experience you had making a change. It does not matter if you choose something that worked well or something that did not work at all. In fact, sometimes the most powerful lessons come from what did not work. As you think about that experience, ask yourself these questions:

- What change did I attempt to make?
- What motivated me to make that change?
- What helped me?
- What got in my way?
- What kind of support was helpful to me?
- What kind of support was not helpful?
- What did I learn about myself as a result of this experience?

As you think about your answers to these questions, you may realize that all you needed to do was make up your mind and you could do it. Or you may have found that external support was important for you. Learning about yourself from your past experiences and considering what helped and hindered you can be a good starting point for making changes.

Bear in mind that there may be a key difference between your past experience with making changes and diabetes. After all, you did not choose to have diabetes or pre-diabetes. You may feel that the changes you are now considering are being imposed on you, while more than likely, the changes you made in the past were your idea. But remember that you do have choices in the way you manage your diabetes. Even though you may feel that your health care team and other people around you are trying to change you, choosing to make changes is still up to you. You are choosing to make them *for yourself*, and they are an essential part of taking charge of your diabetes. Your commitment is critical to your success.

Research has shown that people are more likely to succeed when they first set a long-term goal and then set short-term goals as steps toward reaching it. There are five equally important steps in this process:

1. Define the problem.
2. Recognize your feelings.
3. Choose a goal.
4. Make a plan to reach the goal.
5. Evaluate its outcome.

The information we discussed in the earlier chapters provided a foundation for working through these steps.

DEFINE THE PROBLEM

The first step is to define the problem. A clear definition will lead you to a clear solution. Some people first choose things that are easy for them to do, while others prefer to start with the most challenging issues. The important thing is that you need to be the one who makes the choices and sets the priorities. The following questions can help you begin to think about which problem you wish to address first.

- What is it like for me to live with diabetes?
- What is my greatest concern?
- What is the hardest thing in caring for my diabetes?
- What makes it so hard for me?
- When I think about this problem, what comes to mind?

You may think you already know exactly what the problem is. But often what you believe the problem to be is really only a symptom. If your plan addresses only the symptoms, it becomes like the carnival game, Whac-a-Mole, where you hit the mole into one hole, only to find it popping up from another.

For example, perhaps you identify your problem as sticking with your meal plan. As you think about this, you realize that it is a struggle for you to stop snacking after dinner. The question to ask yourself is "why?" Suppose your answer is that your family members eat at that time, and it is hard for you not to join them. Again, ask yourself "why?" Is it because you feel left out? Is it a family ritual you have always shared? Or is it because they urge you to join them? If the answer is because you feel left out, you may choose to eat something else that will help rather than hinder your efforts to reach your blood sugar and other targets. If your answer is that this is part of your family's routine or that they urge you to join them, then the solution may be different. You may just need to let them know how pressured you feel. If you figure out that you eat because you feel tired in the evening due to stress at work, you may want to think of another way to handle your stress. As you can see, you need clarity and specificity in order to come up with a solution that works.

Keep asking yourself "why" until you get to the heart of the problem. A big clue that

— Marti Speaks —

A woman in one of my classes once told us that since her husband had taken over cooking dinner, she was eating too many starchy vegetables. She chose as a short-term goal to eat more non-starchy vegetables the following week. When she came back to class and I asked how things went, she told us that she was not able to increase her intake of non-starchy vegetables. As she identified strategies she had tried—buying cut-up carrots and celery, buying greens to try a new lower-fat recipe, and prepared salads—I kept asking why each of them did not work. Then the answer dawned on her. She smiled and said, "Since my husband took over the cooking, I have lost twenty pounds by staying out of the kitchen—I am not going back in there for any reason!" ■

the problem has not been completely or correctly identified is that the solution does not work. If this happens, try not to get discouraged, but keep asking "why" until you are clear about the real reason this is a problem for you.

RECOGNIZE YOUR FEELINGS

The second phase is to identify how you feel about the problem. One reason we have focused so much on the emotional side of diabetes in this book is that our feelings have such a strong influence on our behavior. Diabetes is no longer thought of as just a physical problem. If we feel angry and depressed about an issue, it is difficult to think of a solution or take steps to address it. For example, if you feel angry because your family eats ice cream in the evenings, guilty when you join them, and left out when you do not, your anger may cause you either to join them anyway or feel resentful when you pass up the ice cream. Your anger and resentment will often be expressed at other times and in other ways.

Many people believe that there is nothing they can do to change the way they feel. While this is true to some extent, you can influence your feelings by reframing your thoughts. For example, suppose you feel that having diabetes is an unfair burden. What causes you to feel that way? Are there other ways to think about it? Your answers may give you the insight you need to reframe your thoughts, which in turn may help you alter your feelings and behavior. If you feel that you can never make changes because you have failed so often in the past, reminding yourself of what you have now learned from reading this book may increase your confidence.

Many people have difficulty knowing or expressing their feelings. If this is true for you, thinking about the following questions might help. Your answers to these questions can also help you reframe your thoughts.

- How do I feel about my problem?
- What are my thoughts about this problem?
- How will I feel if things do not change?
- How will I feel if things do change?

- How is this issue affecting my ability to enjoy my life?
- What would help me to think differently about this issue?

If you have trouble identifying your feelings, another idea to try is to write a story about your problem. Reading what you have written can help you think more clearly about the problem, your feelings, and whether you are truly prepared to take action to change the situation.

CHOOSE A GOAL

The next step is to identify what you want to accomplish. This is your long-term goal. There are several considerations that may help you clarify it. These questions will also help you understand your motivation for making a change and the importance of a particular goal for you. Once again, you are the only one who can decide whether the outcome will be worth your effort. If you do not believe that it is worthwhile, you will have a hard time staying motivated and sticking with it.

- What do I really want?
- How does the situation or problem that I have identified need to change so I can feel better about it?
- What will I gain if I make this change? What will I give up?
- What will I gain if I do not make this change? What will I give up?
- On a scale of 1 to 10, with 10 being extremely important, how important is this goal to me?
- On a scale of 1 to 10, with 10 being fully confident, how confident do I feel that I can reach my goal?
- Am I ready and willing to take action to reach my goal?
- What needs to happen for me to get what I want?
- What do I need to do?
- Given the reality of my situation and my feelings about this problem, what can I do?

One way to think about willpower is that it equals the level of importance you place on the goal plus the level of confidence you have in your ability to accomplish it. If a goal is important to you and you feel confident that you can reach it, you are more likely to start and continue. If when you think about the score you would give to importance and confidence—on a scale of 1 to 10—and you find that you rate them less than 6 or 7, think about what would have to change for you to raise those numbers. If your answer is that nothing could raise them, it may make sense to choose a different problem or area to tackle. On the other hand, if your rating for either of those questions is 8 or 9, think about what could potentially cause this number to go down. That might help you to identify some negative influences you might encounter that could cause the goal to be less important or lower your confidence. If you feel confident but do not think that the problem is very important, or it is important but you are not very confident you can reach your goal, focus on strategies to increase your confidence or the level of importance before you begin working on it.

MAKE A PLAN TO REACH THE GOAL

You may be tempted to choose a goal without thinking about what you will do to reach it. There are many people who have wanted to lose the same ten pounds for several years but have never done it. Choosing a goal is almost always easier than getting a start towards achieving it.

There are different ways to reach most goals. If your goal is weight loss, you could start by exercising more, eating less fat, cutting out certain foods altogether, or decreasing your portions of high-calorie foods. It is often helpful to brainstorm a list of ideas for reaching your goal. Write everything down, no matter how far-fetched it might seem. Include things that you have tried before: those that worked and those that did not. Your experience might be different this time around.

Review your list and pick one idea. Then identify one step you can take to get started. Be as specific as you can when choosing the step you will take. For example, you might decide that you will eat one sandwich and an apple instead of two sandwiches for lunch four days this week. If, on the other hand, your strategy for losing weight is to be more physically active, you might decide to walk for fifteen minutes during your lunch break three days this week. It is easier to accomplish your goals and evaluate the results when you are clear about exactly what you will do.

You are likely to be more successful if you begin slowly and set a realistic goal. Focus on things you can do that will help you work toward the goal, not on the goal itself. For example, you may not always have total control over your weight, but you do have control over deciding what to eat or whether to exercise. Choosing a step that focuses on your behavior is likely to be more effective than deciding to lose five pounds. Starting with one step allows you to achieve some success, and success builds confidence. Just like in a football game, where it often takes three or four tries to make a first down, you lose weight one meal at a time and lower your blood sugar level one day at a time. Ask yourself these questions as you make your plan:

- What are some ideas I have about strategies that might work?
- What have I tried in the past?
- Why do I think it worked or did not?
- What are some steps I can take to bring myself closer to where I want to be?
- What do I need to do to get started?
- What one thing will I do this week to begin to move toward my goal?
- What is the likelihood that I will do this?

EVALUATE THE OUTCOME

The final step is to experiment with your plan and evaluate the results: the "Es" in the LIFE steps. We call this an experiment because most people need to try several things to figure out what will work best for them. Plus, with an experiment, you always learn something—even when it does not work out as you hoped. In fact, some of the greatest advances in science have occurred when the experiment actually failed. As Henry Ford once said, "Failure is the opportunity to start over with a lot more information."

The question to ask yourself is not whether your experiment worked, but what you learned in the process. Along with focusing on what you learned, some or all of the following questions will help you to evaluate your experiment:

- What would I do the same way next time? What would I do differently?
- What barriers did I encounter? What ideas do I have for overcoming those barriers?
- How do I feel about what I accomplished?
- Was I able to do more or less than I thought? Why?
- Is this still an area on which I want to work?
- What did I learn about myself by doing this experiment?
- Did I learn things about the type of support I need or want?
- What did I learn about how I feel about this problem?
- What did I learn about how important this is to me or how much I value making a change?

MOVING FORWARD

Once you have evaluated your experiment, take time to reward yourself. Be sure to recognize your efforts, no matter what the outcome. Some people find that giving themselves a verbal "pat on the back" is enough while others choose a more tangible reward, such as taking the time to do something they enjoy. The important thing is to applaud your efforts. Recognizing your hard work helps keep you motivated and gives you confidence that you will be able to make further changes.

You are now ready to formulate a new plan, choose another experiment, continue to do what you are doing, or add to the number of times you will do what you chose. If you hit a snag, go back to the beginning of the LIFE process and think through the steps. Your long-term goals may have changed or your level of commitment may be different. At the end of this Chapter there is a summary of all of the steps we have discussed to guide you through this process.

As you continue to try new experiments and evaluate their results, you will learn

A Special Note for Family and Friends

One of the hardest things for family members and friends is to watch their loved ones make decisions that they may not agree with. It is common to be critical or think, "If I were the one with diabetes, I would do more or do better." Although it is true that people with diabetes have to be the final decision makers, their decisions will affect you and your future, and can be a major source of frustration and disagreement. Once again, communication is critical to handling this issue. Realize that attempting to change or control another person adds to the tension and usually causes him or her to become more resistant to your ideas, not less. Instead, try to understand your loved one's decisions and voice your concerns in a caring way. Instead of criticizing or telling him or her what they should do, ask how you can help. Let your loved one know that you care and only want what is best for both of you. ■

more about yourself, your strengths, and what is important to you. You will gain more power over your diabetes and your life.

YOUR LIFE PLAN FOR MANAGING YOUR DIABETES

The following is a summary for you to consider as you formulate, experiment with, and evaluate your self-management plan.

1. **Learn** all you can about diabetes and yourself
2. **Identify** your three guiding principles:
    a) What role do you want to play in the design of your self-management plan?
    b) How much flexibility do you want or need in your plan?
    c) What are your targets for:
    Blood sugar
    A1C
    Blood pressure
    Cholesterol
    Weight

3. **Formulate** your plan:
   Which strategies will you use to reach your targets?
4. **Experiment** with and **Evaluate** your plan:
   What is the problem?
   How do you feel about this issue?
   What is your goal for this issue?
   What step will you take to accomplish your goal? Be sure your step is specific, measurable and doable.
   How did it work?
   What did you learn?
   What is your next step?

Part III: Now What?

CHAPTER 9:
Staying the Course

We wrote this book about the reality of diabetes: the practical challenges of managing diabetes and fitting it into your life. That is why we have called our method the LIFE plan. The LIFE plan provides you with the fundamental roadmap for taking charge of your diabetes as only *you* can.

While it would be nice to think that you now know everything you need to manage your diabetes for the rest of your life, this is probably not the case. Caring for diabetes is a lifelong process, as is learning about it—particularly about *your* diabetes.

Knowing what you want to do is not the same as always being able to do it. You learn by trying and succeeding, and by failing and trying again. You are likely to encounter obstacles and challenges along the way. It takes more than talent and desire to reach your goals.

Along with knowing how to manage your diabetes and make changes in your life, you can learn additional skills that will help you as you go: facing challenges, managing stress, finding support, gaining confidence, and staying psyched.

Most of us use these skills to some extent every day at work, at home, or at school. You may have been doing these things for so long that they are automatic. But surprisingly, most people do not think about applying them when it comes to managing an illness. The secret to taking charge of your diabetes is to use the inner strengths and skills you already have, while discovering new ones as you go forward into the future.

COPING WITH CHALLENGES

No matter how much you want your diabetes to go away, there is no cure at this time. Even if you have pre-diabetes and can bring your blood sugar level into the normal range, you are still at risk for diabetes as you grow older, especially if you become less vigilant about your weight or physical activity.

As you begin to make choices and changes, it is likely that you will encounter some obstacles along the way. Some of these may be small and easily resolved while others may take a great deal of work. No matter how large or small the obstacle, however, there are always choices to make in dealing with it.

In our experiences, we have seen a variety of reactions. Some people choose to take an "ostrich" approach and bury their heads in the sand. They ignore their diabetes or spend a lot of time wishing it would go away.

Others fight against their diabetes or try to outsmart it. This response is often fueled by anger and can be a reaction to feeling that their health care team or family is trying to manage their lives. They try to regain control by rebelling against the advice they get. When they spend a lot of effort reacting to other people, however, they are in reality giving others more control over their lives, not less. Instead of doing what they really want to do, they use all of their energy to reject doing what they think others want them to do.

Another option is to cope with your diabetes. Some people think of coping as passive, and you may feel negatively about the word or the concept. However, coping is actually an active process. Coping requires a conscious decision to make the best of the situation and take charge of your response.

There are a variety of ways that people cope with difficult situations. Diabetes is not likely to be the first or last major challenge you will encounter. Think about how you coped with difficulties in the past. Would any of the strategies you used also help you deal with your diabetes?

STRESS MANAGEMENT

We all have stress in our lives. Diabetes adds more stress, and some people find it harder to handle their everyday stresses once they have diabetes. It is as though they spend all of their energy managing it. Because stress can have a negative effect on both your blood sugar levels and the overall quality of your life, finding new and more effective ways to handle it is part of taking charge of your diabetes. You have three options for dealing with stress: Change your perception of the event, eliminate or avoid the source of your stress, or learn to deal with the situation.

Stress is not a reality; it is a perception. You perceive different events to be stressful or not based on your beliefs about their importance. All you have to do is observe people in an airport when a flight is cancelled to realize how different responses to stress can be. Some people just get angry, some people sit back and wait for the airline to solve the problem, and others actively try to find another flight.

While we cannot always control the events in our lives, we can choose how we respond to them. One strategy for handling stress is to make a conscious decision about how you will respond. To put things into a more manageable perspective, you might try asking yourself, "What is the worst thing that could happen as a result of this event?"

Another approach is to think about the things in your life that are stressful. Often these drain your energy and prevent you from fully enjoying life. One option is to figure out which stresses you can eliminate. If you find that certain situations cause you to feel stressed, try to avoid them as often as you can. Initially, avoiding some of these situations may in itself be stressful; for example, asking someone else to take on a task you have done in the past. It takes time and practice to learn to say no. Other people might not do things the same way or as well as you do, but they usually work out just fine.

There are stresses you just cannot eliminate, so it helps to have a plan to manage them. One way is through physical activity, since exercise increases the level of endorphins—the "feel good" hormones. Endorphins help counteract the effects of stress hormones, both physically and emotionally. Some people find meditation, prayer, or reading inspirational messages to be calming. Others are helped by a good listener or writing down their feelings and problems.

Drinking alcohol and smoking are ways some people deal with stress. Such a response may make them feel better temporarily, but does not really solve the problem and can ultimately do more harm than good. Eating is another common way to handle stress. There is nothing inherently wrong with eating when stressed; the issue is what we eat and how much. Most of us do not think of cooking a pot of broccoli to eat when we are stressed! Questions to ask yourself about the way you cope with stress are:

- Did it help?
- Did I feel better or worse?
- If I felt better, for how long?
- Did I feel better or worse the next morning?
- Did my approach cause additional stress or relieve it?

In reality, if we had no stress in our lives we would probably be bored. Holidays, vacations, and other celebrations can be somewhat stressful, but are also enjoyable. They take us out of the routine of our lives and give us satisfaction as well. Just as with other aspects of diabetes management, the trick is to find the right balance of positive and negative stressors in your life.

FINDING SUPPORT

Research has shown that people do better managing their diabetes when they have the support of their family and friends. This does not mean that family and friends manage it for you, but that they are there to celebrate your achievements with you and listen when you are feeling down.

The best way to get the support you need is to ask for it. People who care about you usually want to be helpful, but they may not always know how. Remember that they are probably worried about you and think that their actions are supportive. But since you are the one who needs support, you get to decide what actually helps. The first step is to figure out what you want and need. Do you want your family to ask how you are coping? Would it help if they ate similar food or exercised with you? Do you want them to ask about your blood sugar readings or wait until you tell them your number?

Once you decide what you want, you need to let your family members know. This can be a tricky conversation to have. Using "I" statements usually works better than making critical statements. For example, you could say, "I know you are worried about me and I appreciate your concern, but I am embarrassed when you call attention to what I am eating in front of other people. It would help more if you listened to me talk about my diabetes."

Sometimes your family and friends are not able or willing to support you. Just as you have the right to ask for what you need, they have the right to say no. This is not a negative reflection on either you or them; it is simply a fact. If you believe that support will help, you may want to find another way to get it: your health care team or perhaps your clergy. Many communities have diabetes support groups. There, you can talk with others who often have the same problems and concerns as you and understand what you are going through. If you feel that you would benefit from this, ask your diabetes educator if there is a support group in your area.

GAINING CONFIDENCE AND STAYING PSYCHED

In football, it is not just about the plays. There is the emotional side of the game as well. Quarterbacks need to believe in themselves and stay psyched, even when the going gets tough. So do you.

One of the ways to gain confidence is to recognize the progress you are making with each step you take toward your goal. Another is to remember to congratulate yourself upon each accomplishment. If you often think negative thoughts about your abilities, it is easy to lose confidence. If you think you will never be able to lose weight, you are probably correct. If you tell yourself that you can do it, you probably can. Although it may sound simplistic, reframing your thoughts and giving yourself positive messages can really work to build your confidence. As you become more confident, you are more likely to reach your goals, which will boost your self-confidence even more.

Part of being in charge of your diabetes is learning how to use your emotions instead of letting them defeat you. For example, one way to think about diabetes is to consider it a complete disaster. In many ways, that is a true statement. Another way to think about diabetes is that it is a powerful motivator to take charge of your health and your life. This is also true. If diabetes feels like a burden, try reminding yourself that you can live a good life and still take care of your diabetes.

If these statements do not ring true for you, try reframing your own thoughts in a way that does. Many people find it helpful to write down their feelings so that they can examine them more closely. Writing down negative thoughts can help release them. By reading what you have written, you may be able to identify your struggles more clearly and figure out other ways to think about diabetes and its impact on your life. Not only is writing things down a way to ease your emotional distress, but reading what you have written can sometimes help you discover a solution to what seemed like a hopeless situation. Writing gives you the opportunity to reflect, and through reflection, to gain insight.

Our thoughts affect our feelings and how we behave. Changing your thoughts can help you feel more confident and more empowered to take charge of your diabetes.

GET INVOLVED

One of the ways to gain support and channel some of your negative feelings into positive action is to get involved in causes or activities that are important to you. There are several organizations that work to benefit people with diabetes. The largest of these are the American Diabetes Association (ADA) and the Juvenile Diabetes Research Foundation (JDRF). The mission of the ADA is to prevent and cure diabetes and to improve the lives of all people affected by diabetes. The JDRF is dedicated to finding a cure for type 1 diabetes and its complications. Diabetes organizations offer a variety of activities including fundraising events such as walks and bike rides, advocacy efforts, camps, and educational or support programs. By becoming involved, you can help yourself and meet other people who share your interest and concerns, and at the same time do something positive for others. To start, pick the activity which appeals most to you.

There are other ways to get involved as well. If you are already part of a community or religious organization, there may be ways to spread awareness about diabetes in and through that organization. Although it takes time and energy to volunteer, most people feel that they gain more than they give.

LOOKING TO THE FUTURE

Research in diabetes continues to progress at a promising pace. In fact, many of the therapies, recommendations, and strategies included in this book are based on what has been learned through recent research efforts.

There are five main areas in which research efforts are concentrated at this time: a cure, prevention and treatment of complications, medications and other therapies, technology and translation.

The Search for a Cure

Efforts to find a cure for both type 1 and type 2 diabetes are ongoing and intensive. Early results from transplanting islet cells in people with type 1 diabetes have been promising. However, much work remains to be done before this therapy will be widely available. Stem cells are also an area of intense research interest in the quest for a cure.

Complications Research

The very real threat of developing complications is a serious concern for most people with diabetes. Although research has shown the benefits of intensive blood sugar management to prevent these complications, they continue to occur despite the best efforts of patients and their providers. Research efforts today are focused on better therapies to prevent complications from occurring and to treat them when they do. Current therapies for complications are better at relieving symptoms and slowing their progress than past therapies, but once again, more work needs to be done.

Medications and Other Therapies

Although there are more options and better therapies for treating diabetes than ever before, scientists continue to search for even better ones. The new synthetic hormones are an example of these efforts. Research continues to discover other methods of treating both type 1 and type 2 diabetes, as well as pre-diabetes, and to find new medications that will work even more effectively than what is currently available.

Technology

As in other fields, technology is helping advance the care of diabetes. Continuous glucose monitors and inhaled insulin are examples of how technology has been applied to the treatment of diabetes. Researchers continue to try to find better ways to administer insulin without needles. In addition, there is a great deal of interest in creating both external and internal "closed loop systems" where a continuous glucose monitor could communicate with an insulin pump to provide the precise level of insulin needed to manage blood sugar levels. This would function much as the pancreas does in people without diabetes. Although it would not be a cure, it would involve a great deal less decision-making and trial and error than our current therapies.

Translational Research

Translational research is taking what is learned in the laboratory or in controlled clinical trials and applying it to the real world. Many clinical recommendations about the management of blood sugar, blood pressure, and lipid levels are based on translating the results of clinical trials into practice.

Another area of translational research is to understand more about how people with diabetes feel about their illness, how they manage it on a daily basis, how they make changes in their health behaviors, and how health professionals can work more effectively with their patients. The DAWN (Diabetes Attitudes, Wishes and Needs) study is an example of a large scientific study designed to determine how people with diabetes respond emotionally and manage it, and what strategies are effective in supporting their efforts. Many of the strategies recommended in this book, such as empowerment, are based on translational research findings about how people with diabetes learn and make changes. Efforts continue in this area, as do research projects to learn more about depression, quality of life, and coping.

You may see ads in your local newspaper or on TV or hear ads on the radio recruiting patients with diabetes to participate in research. These studies generally undergo rigorous review so that your rights and safety are protected. Consider getting involved. It is a great way to learn about and receive the latest in diabetes care and contribute to others who have, or are at risk for, diabetes.

Funding

No discussion of research could be fair or complete without some mention of the many funding sources that make diabetes research possible. The federal government, through the National Institutes of Health, the Centers for Disease Control and Prevention, the Department of Defense, and various other agencies, provides hundreds of millions of diabetes research dollars every year. These expenditures are not guaranteed, however, and it is in the best interest of all persons affected by diabetes—patients, family members, friends, and business associates—to do whatever they can to keep those funds flowing by letting their elected representatives know of their interest in this important area of research.

This is not just a government function, however. Private sector companies in the pharmaceutical and medical device industries are continually searching for new and better therapies and equipment to help in the treatment of diabetes and its complications. Major universities and charitable organizations like the ADA, the JDRF, and a host of public and private foundations are constantly raising funds to finance diabetes research projects. Again, by becoming involved in the activities of these organizations, you can go a long way towards supporting needed research achievements.

• • •

We have heard people describe diabetes as a heavy weight that they always carry with them. Our goal for this book is to help lighten that load by making your life with diabetes easier and less of a burden. As you reach the end of this book, we hope that you have begun to develop a more positive and helpful plan for approaching your life with diabetes, and that you are finding the motivation you need to tackle it. This motivation comes from creating a workable overall strategy and making informed choices and changes. True motivation comes from within. Others can inspire and support your efforts, but only you can create the motivation you need for a lifetime of diabetes care. It *is* all about you.

Think LIFE.

A Special Note for Family and Friends

Living with diabetes day in and day out is hard work and can be wearing for people who have it and those around them. There will probably be times when you wish that you could take a vacation from your loved one's diabetes. Because it is a lifetime condition, your continued love and support are important for sustaining motivation and commitment. Do not be discouraged by particular choices or outcomes. It is what happens most of the time that counts. Confidence in the overall plan and in your loved one's decisions will go a long way toward ensuring the best results. ■

Appendix 1

GLOSSARY OF TERMS

A1C: A measurement of average blood sugar levels over the prior two to three months. Recommended A1C levels are discussed on page 81.

Amylin: A hormone made in the **pancreas** that together with **insulin** helps keep blood sugar levels from going too high after meals.

Basal level: The steady low level of **insulin** used to regulate blood sugar levels between meals.

Beta cells: The cells of the **pancreas** that manufacture and release **insulin**.

Bolus: A burst or extra shot of **insulin** to cover increases in blood sugar at mealtime.

Carbohydrates: Another word for sugar and starch in the diet. Carbohydrates are broken down into glucose during digestion and are the body's main source of energy.

CDE (certified diabetes educator): A health professional who has passed a national exam in diabetes education.

Cholesterol: A waxy, fat-like substance in the blood. **LDL**, or low-density lipoprotein, is the "bad" or "lousy" kind of cholesterol that deposits fat in the blood vessels. **HDL**, or high-density lipoprotein, is the "good" or "helpful" kind of cholesterol that removes fat deposits from the blood vessels.

DAWN: The Diabetes Attitudes Wishes and Needs Study that assessed psychological health, patient provider communication, access to team care, and access to effective therapy. More than 5,100 people with type 1 and type 2 diabetes and 3,800 physicians and nurses from thirteen countries participated in this international study.

DCCT: The Diabetes Control and Complications Trial that demonstrated that keeping blood sugar levels closer to normal helps reduce the risk of complications for people with type 1 diabetes.

DPP: The Diabetes Prevention Program that demonstrated that a 5 to 7 percent weight loss and thirty minutes of exercise five days a week reduced the incidence of diabetes among people at risk.

DPP-IV Inhibitors (dipeptidyl peptidase IV inhibitors) Enhances the action of the incretin hormones, which stimulate the release of insulin from the pancreas and block the release of glucagons from the liver. This extends the action of insulin while suppressing the release of glucagon.

Endocrinologist: A physician specializing in the study of insulin and other hormones.

Erectile Dysfunction: The inability to have or maintain an erection; also called impotence.

Formulary: A health insurance company's published list of the medicines that are approved for coverage.

Glucose: A form of sugar that serves as fuel for the body.

GLP-1 (glucagon-like peptide 1): A hormone made by the cells lining the gut that helps the pancreas to secrete more insulin and improves the ability of the body to use carbohydrates.

Hyperglycemia: A condition in which there is too much sugar in the bloodstream. This can cause tiredness, irritability, hunger, weight loss, dryness, thirst, increased urination, and blurred vision. If not treated, continued **hyperglycemia** can result in coma and death.

Hypoglycemia: A condition in which there is too little sugar (less than 70 mg/dl or 3.9 mmol/l) in the bloodstream. This can cause sweatiness, dizziness, hunger, weakness, irritability, and confusion. If not treated immediately by ingesting sugar, **hypoglycemia** can result in coma and death.

Impaired Glucose Tolerance (IGT): Blood sugar levels that are higher than normal levels, but not high enough to be considered diagnostic of diabetes. Also called pre-diabetes. A fasting blood sugar between 100 (5.6 mmol/l) and 125 mg/dl (6.9 mmol/l), and a reading of between 140 and 199 mg/dl (7.8 and 11.0 mmol/l)two hours after a meal is considered pre-diabetes. Two fasting blood sugar readings of 126 (7.0 mmol/l) or higher or readings of 200 mg/dl (11.1 mmol/l) or higher two hours after a meal is diagnostic of diabetes.

Insulin: A hormone produced by the **beta cells** in the **pancreas**. It is necessary for moving sugar from the bloodstream into the body's cells, where it can be used for energy.

Ketoacidosis: A severe condition caused by a lack of **insulin**. Symptoms include high blood sugar, low blood pressure, ketones in the urine, dehydration, and breath with a sweet fruity odor.

Ketosis: The presence in the urine of ketones, which are chemicals produced when the body breaks down fat for fuel.

Nephropathy: Damage to the small blood vessels in the kidneys.

Neuropathy: Nerve damage.

Pancreas: The gland in the body that produces **insulin** and other hormones used to regulate blood sugar levels.

Retinopathy: Damage to the small blood vessels in the eyes that can lead to blindness if untreated.

Triglycerides: A type of fat carried in the bloodstream.

UKPDS: The United Kingdom Prospective Diabetes Study that demonstrated that keeping blood sugar levels closer to normal helps reduce the risk of complications for people with type 2 diabetes.

Appendix 2

RESOURCES

You may find the following resources helpful.

ORGANIZATIONS
American Association of Diabetes Educators
100 W. Monroe Street, Suite 400
Chicago, IL 60603
1-800-338-3633
www.aadenet.org

American Diabetes Association
1701 N. Beauregard Street
Alexandria, VA 22311
1-800-342-2383
www.diabetes.org

American Dietetic Association
120 S. Riverside Plaza, Suite 2000
Chicago, IL 60606
1-800-877-1600
www.eatright.org
Juvenile Diabetes Research Foundation
    International
120 Wall Street, 19th Floor

New York, NY 10005
1-800-533-2873
www.jdrf.org

National Diabetes Education Program
1 Diabetes Way
Bethesda, MD 20814
www.ndep.nih.gov

Magazines

Diabetes Forecast
American Diabetes Association
P.O. Box 363
Mt. Morris, IL 61054-0363
1-800-342-2383
www.diabetes.org/diabetes-forecast.jsp

Diabetes Self-Management
150 W. 22nd Street
Dept. BIO
New York, NY 10011
1-800-234-0923
www.diabetesselfmanagement.com

Diabetes Explorer
PO Box 432
Oregon, IL 61061-0432
www.diabetes-explorer.com

Diabetes Health
6 School Street
Suite: 160
Fairfax, CA 94930-1650
(800) 234-1218
www.diabeteshealth.com

Diabetes Digest
5 South Myrtle Ave.
Spring Valley, NY 10977
1-845-426-7612
www.diabetesdigest.com

Diabetic Living
5085 NE 17th Street
Des Moines, IA 50313
www.bhg.com

Diabetes America
3 Riverway Suite 825
Houston, TX 77056
830-237-3500
www.diabetesamerica.com/contact.cfm

Countdown
Juvenile Diabetes Research Foundation
   International
120Wall Street, 19th Floor
New York, NY 10005-4001
www.jdrf.org

Diabetes Close Up
Close Concerns, Inc.
One Ferry Building, Suite 255
San Francisco, CA 94111
415-241-9500
www.closeconcerns.com

BOOKS

There are many books available online, at your local bookstore, or from the American Diabetes Association. This is a brief listing of some that we think can be particularly helpful. There are also many cookbooks and menu guides available from the American Diabetes Association and the American Dietetic Association. The American Diabetes Association also publishes a series of short books called "101 Tips..."

American Diabetes Association Complete Guide to Diabetes, 4th edition (Alexandria, VA: American Diabetes Association, 2005)

Carol Guber's Type 2 Diabetes Life Plan by Carol Guber, MS (New York: Broadway Books, 2002)

Conquering Diabetes by Anne L. Peters, MD (New York: Plume, 2005)

Diabesity by Francine R. Kaufman, MD (New York: Bantam, 2005)

Diabetes: A Guide to Living Well, 4th edition, by Gary Arsham, MD, PhD and Ernest Lowe (Alexandria, VA: American Diabetes Association, 2003)

Diabetes: A Practical Guide to Managing Your Health by Rosemary Walker and Jill Rogers (New York: Dorling Kindersley, 2004)

Diabetes A to Z, 5th edition, by the American Diabetes Association (Alexandria, VA: American Diabetes Association, 2003)

Diabetes Burnout: What to Do When You Can't Take It Anymore by William H. Polonsky, PhD, CDE (Alexandria, VA: American Diabetes Association, 1999)

Diabetes on Your Own Terms by Janis Roszler, RD, CDE, LD/N (New York: Marlowe and Co., 2007)

Dr. Gavin's Health Guide for African Americans by James R. Gavin, MD, PhD (Alexandria, VA: Small Steps Press, 2004)

Guide to Raising a Child with Diabetes by Linda Siminerio, RN, PhD, CDE, and Jean Betschart MN, MSN, CPNP, CDE (Alexandria, VA: American Diabetes Association, 2000)

Managing Diabetes Your Way Workbook by Beth Ann Petro Roybal (Berkeley, CA: Ulysses Press, 2005)

Psyching Out Diabetes: A Positive Approach to Your Negative Emotions, 3rd edition, by Richard R. Rubin, PhD, CDE (Los Angeles: McGraw-Hill, 1999)

Taking Control of Your Diabetes, 2nd edition, by Steven V. Edelman, MD (Caddo, OK: Professional Communications, 2001)

The Diabetes Problem-Solver: Quick Answers to Your Questions About Treatment and Self-Care, 2nd edition, by Nancy Touchette, PhD (Alexandria, VA: American Diabetes Association, 2006)

The Diabetes Travel Guide, 2nd edition, by Davida Kruger, MSN, RN, BC-ADM (Alexandria, VA: American Diabetes Association, 2007)

The First Year—Type 2 Diabetes: An Essential Guide for the Newly Diagnosed by Gretchen

Becker (New York: Marlowe and Co., 2001)

The "I Hate to Exercise" Book for People with Diabetes by Charlotte Hayes, MMSc, MS, RD, CDE (Alexandria, VA: American Diabetes Association, 2001)

The Secrets of Living and Loving with Diabetes by Janis Roszler, RD, CDE, LD/N, William H. Polonsky, PhD, CDE, Steven V. Edelman, MD (Chicago: Surrey Books, 2004)

Type 2 Diabetes for Beginners by Phyllis Barrier, MS, RD (Alexandria, VA: American Diabetes Association, 2005)

The Uncomplicated Guide to Diabetes Complications, 3rd edition, by Marvin Levin, MD. Michael Pfeifer, MD, CDE (Alpharetta, GA: American Diabetes Association, 2007)